Stressed Out

About Drug Interactions

Sheri Lynn Jacobson, MS, APRN

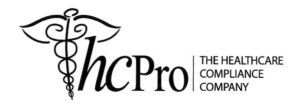

*hc*Pro | THE HEALTHCARE COMPLIANCE COMPANY

Stressed Out About Drug Interactions is published by HCPro, Inc.

Copyright 2007 HCPro, Inc.

ISBN 978-1-57839-974-1

Sheri Lynn Jacobson, MS, APRN, Author
Michael Briddon, Associate Editor
Emily Sheahan, Group Publisher
Shane Katz, Cover Designer
Mike Mirabello, Senior Graphic Artist
Susan Darbyshire, Art Director
Jean St. Pierre, Director of Operations
Darren Kelly, Books Production Supervisor
Audrey Doyle, Copyeditor

Cover illustration by Graham Smith, ArtMasters

Advice given is general. Readers should consult professional counsel for specific legal, ethical, or clinical questions.

Arrangements can be made for quantity discounts. For more information, contact

HCPro, Inc.
P.O. Box 1168
Marblehead, MA 01945
Telephone: 800/650-6787 or 781/639-1872
Fax: 781/639-2982
E-mail: *customerservice@hcpro.com*

Visit the Stressed Out Web site for more information: *www.stressedoutnurses.com*

Dedication

"Take not one day for granted, for this day we know not what tomorrow will bring." Author unknown

I dedicate this book in memory of my father, Samuel J. Jacobson, who valued service to others his entire life, and to my best friend "Sal," whose life yet honored was much too short.

Contents

Part I: Writing the script: The basics about drugs

How to use this book

What if there was a book that explained complex nursing topics in an easy-to-understand manner and in an accessible format? That's the premise behind the Stressed Out…series. Solid references with a bit of a sense of humor and the understanding that a lighthearted approach to learning makes the whole thing more enjoyable.

To help you navigate through the book, you will find the following icons highlighting a particular passage:

 Don't forget: A little reminder about something of importance.

 Ask: This icon directs you to search for further information from an individual or organization.

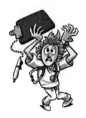 **Don't panic:** Take a deep breath and relax. Here is a little reassurance.

 Fact: Highlights a statistic or truth.

Tip: A bit of inside information, a hint, or helpful advice.

 Watch out: Word to the wise; this is a warning.

 Click: This icon refers you to a helpful Web site, where you may find further information on the topic.

Happy Nursing! Now you're ready to get started.

About the author

Sheri Lynn Jacobson, MS, APRN

Sheri Lynn Jacobson, MS, APRN, is currently a full-time assistant professor in nursing at Winston-Salem State University in Winston-Salem, NC.

She earned her Master of Science of Nursing from Syracuse University as an Adult Nurse Practitioner with a specialty in primary care and a post master's certificate in Web development from East Carolina University. She has been a pediatric nurse for 22 years and a nursing educator for the past 18 years. Her main research interests include integrative medicine, pharmacology, pediatrics, critical thinking in nursing, and online education. Her teaching subjects include pharmacology in nursing, drug math, health assessment, pediatrics, nursing research, and issues and trends in nursing. She has developed both online and Web-assisted nursing courses.

She enjoys serving as a book reviewer and has reviewed titles for HCPro, Thomson Delmar Learning, and Lippincott Williams & Wilkins.

Acknowledgments

I am grateful to have the opportunity to create such an important book to assist nursing students and new graduates with essential pharmacological concepts regarding drug interactions and medication safety. I hope this book will inspire others to take the step to be safe which in reality takes no greater amount of time.

I would like to express my appreciation to my editors Rebecca Hendren and Mike Briddon for their professional support and guidance. Mike Briddon has especially been a guide and support through the entire process of this book.

I want to thank you the reader for recognizing the importance of this work. I encourage you to be a role model for other nurses and health professionals and an advocate for client safety.

Finally, in honoring the words of Helen Keller: *"The Best and most Beautiful Things in the World cannot be Seen or even Touched. They must be Felt with the Heart."* Perform all your endeavors with your heart, and you will always demonstrate the best of who you are.

Introduction

It's Your Movie!

Let's cast you in your own story . . . the story of your safe practice when administering medications and protecting your clients from potential drug interactions and adverse drug events. You can become the heroes and heroines of your own movies in the healthcare arena . . .

We all enjoy getting caught up in a good movie with an interesting plot, compelling characters, moving action, and an intriguing ending. So why can't learning be as enticing and intriguing as a good movie—one that leaves you thinking about it again and again and reliving the most exciting parts? Learning can be just that and *more*.

In an age of technological explosion and a generation that has grown up with high-tech computers, gaming, and entertainment, it is a challenge for educators to make learning inviting and irresistible. But learning is exciting. In nursing, there are constant technological advancements, information systems and practice applications for safety, communication, and convenience, and performances demonstrating expert care with clients.

This book is a story, an evolution, just like a movie, where the plot unfolds and grows as the nurse becomes involved in the process. The twists and turns follow the pharmacological concepts. The peaks are recognizing potential hidden dangers within the world of drug administration for the client, and the ending where the nurse analyzes the story into parts and wholes that can be applied in daily nursing practice.

Stressed Out About Drug Interactions will help you safely and successfully perform your drug administration duties wherever you are with confidence reflective of evidence-based practice, critical thought, and expert execution.

This book will take you forward in your journey, with the following goals:

- Analysis of pharmacological concepts related to drug action

- Identification of pitfalls to avoid in practice when administering drugs

- Guidance toward expert knowledge for safe practice applications

- Recommendations for preparation regarding drug research

- Utilizing drug resources regarding drug interactions, while still economizing on time

- Reviewing commonly administered drugs and their potential interactions

So let's begin. It's time to give our attention to our evolving movie. Is everyone ready? Please, quiet on the set. We're ready to roll!

Part One

Before any great movie goes to production, we first must write the script. In this section, we'll focus on the basics—from pharmacokinetics and pharmacodynamics to some essential drug calculations. Once we've introduced the main characters of our plot, drug interactions will take center stage.

Chapter 1

Lights, camera, drug interaction

When the director yells "lights, camera, action," all the key people involved—producers, directors, actors, and crew members—begin shooting the movie. Setting the story into motion starts the film.

When a drug enters the body, a similar call to action occurs. Drugs and other chemicals such as hormones, enzymes, proteins, and ions are called to action to interact with cell membranes that switch cellular functions on or off, causing an effect within the body. This effect may or may not be beneficial. A therapeutic effect causes a beneficial response, whereas an adverse effect causes a response that may be more serious and even detrimental to the body. Once a drug enters the body, many key processes are set into motion.

Pharmacokinetics and pharmacodynamics: Let the action begin

Looking through the lens of the camera, the cameraman views the action of the movie. Similarly, studying pharmacokinetic and pharmacodynamic action of drugs facilitates your view of how the body responds to drugs and how drugs affect the body. Pharmacokinetics refers to the processes by which drugs are absorbed, distributed, metabolized, and eliminated by the body. The activity is dynamic and for this reason pharmacodynamics must be considered in exploring the effects drugs have on the body.

The actor masters the craft of acting and becomes a professional performer with accolades and promise for future artistic endeavors. Mastering these pharmacological concepts will afford you, the nurse, accolades in your performance of client care related to drug administration. Let your future endeavors, and your award-winning performance, begin.

The study of drug interactions requires critical thought. Elements of critical thinking include

- problem recognition

- analyzing

- synthesizing

- evidence

- problem solving

- evaluation

 Ask: How do you think your point of view will change as you grow in your understanding and knowledge of drug actions? As you read this book, observe how your point of view about drug interactions changes concerning the care of your clients.

> "To learn, and from time to time to apply what
> one has learned, isn't that a pleasure?"
>
> —Confucius

Chapter 2

Pharmacokinetics: It's relationship time

Pharmacokinetics is the relationship that occurs when a drug enters the bloodstream and activates responses within the body. There are four processes that take place when a drug activates a response within the body. These processes are

- absorption

- distribution

- metabolism

- elimination

Absorption takes center stage

Absorption takes place as soon as the drug is introduced into the body and enters circulation. For example, when a client takes a tablet, it begins dissolving with the help of saliva and further disintegrates within the stomach by gastric secretions before entering the circulation via the bloodstream. The effect of drug action occurs as the medication enters the bloodstream and produces a physiologic effect.

Tip: When dealing with enteric coated tablets, remember they are coated to dissolve in the small intestine, not the stomach where irritation can occur. An example is aspirin, which is very irritating to the stomach. On the other hand, enteric coatings can prevent stomach acid from destroying the medication. Do not crush or remove coating, which destroys the intended protection.

There are many variables that may aid or hinder the absorption of a drug. Variables such as dosage form, route of administration, site of administration, food, other medications, and current condition of the client influence the rate and amount of absorption and, ultimately, the effect(s) produced within the body.

As a nurse, you must consider the hierarchy of absorption and resultant effects according to the form of the medication. Liquids absorb faster than tablets or capsules. Topical medications are dependent upon sites such as skin, mucous membranes, and body surface areas with absorption rates, and extents vary accordingly. Medications are rapidly absorbed intramuscularly and subcutaneously. Muscles have more blood vessels than subcutaneous tissues, so intramuscular administration of medications occurs more rapidly than subcutaneous administration.

The intravenous (IV) method of drug administration is the most rapid route because no absorption is necessary and the effect occurs as soon as the medication enters the bloodstream.

Bioavailability: Is the drug on cue?

An important concept to consider in relation to absorption is bioavailability. Following our earlier filmmaking example, the movie cannot be produced if the actor is in the dressing room or out to lunch. The actor must be available to act. Drugs, similarly, must be available to produce their effects within the body whether they enter directly into the bloodstream or are metabolized in the liver.

A bioavailable drug is only available to the extent of the route and how the drug is characteristically metabolized. Oral medications are less than 100% bioavailable, whereas the IV route is usually 100% bioavailable. Other drugs that are metabolized first in the liver route vary in bioavailability—and would thus be unreliable actors. (We wouldn't want them to miss a cue.)

Some drugs pass through the liver for metabolism more than once, with the first time being considered the hepatic first-pass effect, which has a bioavailability between 20%–60%. Some medications administered orally bypass systemic circulation and pass from the intestinal membranes directly into the liver via the portal vein where metabolism of the drug occurs. Drugs that are metabolized in the liver may have a varying effect and require larger prescribed doses to ensure a therapeutic effect. Factors that affect the bioavailability of drugs include

- route

- drug form

- food

- other drugs

- gastrointestinal mucosa and motility

- hepatic blood flow

- rate of administration

 Watch out: Some drugs when given too rapidly or too frequently can cause toxicity in the client. Check drug references for specific administration time frames and appropriate frequency.

Drug distribution: There are a variety of roles

Now that the drug has entered the body, what happens next? It is distributed throughout the body's intricate network of tissues, where pharmacologic activity occurs through the processes of drug distribution, metabolism, and elimination.

When making a movie, the producer distributes the script to the actors so they will know their lines and can act in the movie. Similarly, drugs must be distributed within the body to cause an effect.

Drug distribution is the process where drugs become available to the body once they travel through body fluids or tissues. How does a drug produce an effect once distributed within the body? Drugs travel through the body fluids, have affinity to cells, and are greatly influenced by protein within the body. Most drugs are bound to protein (albumin) in varying degrees.

Like a lead actress and actor who have a liking for each other in a romantic movie, drugs have an affinity to cells and body tissues. Drugs may have varying degrees of affinity and, for this reason, may be highly, moderately, or lowly protein bound. The amount of drug not bound to protein is considered free drug. This portion of the drug is free to travel within the circulation and produce a physiologic effect on the body. As the free drug is used up within the body, more protein-bound drug is released to continue drug action.

Watch out: When two leading men in the movie have affinity for the leading actress, some kind of high drama is likely to occur—a fight, a duel, a conflict for the lovely lady's love and attention. A toxic effect may occur that could potentially be lethal. The same is true in drug interactions: A toxic effect and drug accumulation may result when two highly protein-bound drugs are administered together. In addition, when a client has a low plasma protein (albumin) level, there are not enough protein-binding sites to which the drug can attach. This results in more free drug traveling within the circulation unbound. This excess free drug initiates drug action and may result in drug overdose and toxic effects. When clients are malnourished, elderly, or have certain health conditions such as kidney or liver dysfunction, they may have abnormally low plasma protein (albumin) levels, which contribute to a higher risk of drug overdose and toxicity.

Don't forget: Always consider the client's potential for drug toxicity when administering any medication. Checking protein-binding potential for all drugs, plasma protein and albumin levels, and current nutritional status can prevent life-threatening toxic effects of drugs for the client.

Metabolism: Breaking it down into smaller parts

For the actor to learn his or her part in the movie, the part must be broken down into scenes and lines so the actor can become the character to deliver the performance. For drugs to be broken down into smaller parts within the body, the process of metabolism must occur. Metabolism occurs within the liver, where drugs are inactivated and are further broken down into metabolites by liver enzymes. Many drugs are lipid soluble. The liver converts lipid-soluble drugs to water-soluble substances for excretion by the kidneys. Metabolites are the active parts of drugs that can cause an increased pharmacological response, especially in clients who have liver dysfunction or diseases. When drug metabolism is decreased, there is an increased likelihood of drug accumulation, which can result in toxicity.

Half the drug it used to be

The half-life of a drug is the time span that it takes for one-half of the drug to be eliminated and is denoted as t $^1/_2$. Drug half-life is affected by both metabolism and elimination, especially with liver and kidney dysfunction. An example of this is when a client has hepatitis (a liver disease), and the half-life is prolonged because less drug is being metabolized. Most drugs go through many half-lives until they are fully eliminated. To illustrate this concept, let's use the example of 650 mg of acetaminophen. With a half-life of three hours (information that can be found in any drug reference), 650 mg of acetaminophen is ingested, then it takes three hours for the first half-life to eliminate half the drug to 325 mg, and then six hours for the second half-life to eliminate an additional 162 mg, and so on. The process is mathematical, and after each three hours, another half of the drug is eliminated.

Half-life for acetaminophen 650 mg

t1/2 NUMBER OF HALF-LIVES	TIME (IN HOURS)	DOSAGE REMAINING (mg)	PERCENT REMAINING
1	3	325	50
2	6	162	25
3	9	81	12.5
4	12	40	6.25
5	15	20	3.1
6	18	10	1.55

Kidneys' role in drug elimination

The kidneys are the main pathway for drug elimination. Drugs are eliminated via the urine. Drug elimination is influenced by urine pH and kidney function. Impaired kidney functioning results in decreases in glomerular filtration rates (GFR), which leads to a reduction of drug elimination. Adverse drug reactions can result from drug accumulation related to abnormal kidney functioning. Drug dosages may need to be reduced in the elderly because kidney function declines due to age, and in young children, who have immature kidneys.

Watch out: You must pay close attention to monitoring kidney lab values (e.g., serum creatinine and BUNs) to safeguard clients against drug overdoses and toxicities due to drug accumulation.

"Not everything that can be counted, counts, and not everything that counts can be counted."

—Albert Einstein

Chapter 3

Cue pharmacodynamics and drugs in motion

The actors cast in a movie must be dynamic so it will be a hit. The study of drugs and their related responses upon the human body is also dynamic.

Pharmacodynamics is the inquiry into the effects that a drug has on cellular physiology partnered with the biochemical reactions caused by the drug's mechanisms of action. Drug responses may be primary or secondary. A primary drug response is when the administered drug causes its intended effect. A secondary drug response, which may happen in addition to the primary drug response, may or may not be beneficial. For example, a primary effect of an antihistamine is decongestion—which would be a desired effect—but a secondary effect could be drowsiness, which would definitely be undesirable when, for example, someone is driving.

Drugs and cells create key interactions

Drugs affect the body by interacting with cellular functioning. These interactions are dependent upon the body's cells and the cells' particular function within the body. Drugs must interact with cellular membranes for a physiological response to be activated. The point where this response occurs is referred to as the receptor site. According to receptor theory, drugs and receptors have a "lock and key" effect, in which the drug substance actually binds to cell membranes. For many drugs, the exact mechanism between cellular functioning and drug interaction may be unknown.

Drugs can affect the functioning of cells by increasing, decreasing, or blocking their activity; replacing cell contents; and assisting with substances being transported across cell membranes. Drug action—or the drug's ability to produce an effect—is dependent upon the affinity, or the attraction, that occurs between the drug and the cell receptor and its intrinsic activity. Two types of responses occur when drugs bind with receptors:

- Agonist

- Antagonist

An agonist response is when a drug interacts with a receptor on a cell and activates drug action. An example of an agonist effect is when acetaminophen is given to a child to reduce a fever. Acetaminophen has antipyretic properties, so-called fever reducing magic, and is commonly used for this purpose. An antagonist response is when the drug blocks the receptor on the cell and prevents a cellular response. When overdoses occur, an antagonist drug such as narcan can be administered to block or counteract the effect of too much narcotic such as morphine sulfate.

Drugs are considered either selective (for specific receptors) or nonselective. In some situations, activity occurs at different receptor sites. Within the body, there are target sites where drugs attach to receptors. Some of these target sites are in the salivary glands, heart, blood vessels, lungs, airways, stomach, intestines, bladder, muscles, lacrimal, and sweat glands. When a drug response is not stimulated by action upon receptors, a response is activated by the stimulation or inhibition of enzymes or hormones.

Potency and efficacy: Is it strong enough to be my drug?

A drug's potency is its strength in producing an effect, whereas a drug's efficacy is measured by its effectiveness in producing therapeutic effects. For example, when a client has a headache, you may have orders to administer acetaminophen or acetaminophen with codeine. Because efficacy refers to a drug's maximum potential for therapeutic effectiveness, you must decide which drug to administer, considering the client's intensity of pain, other drugs the client is taking, and potential side effects when surveying the situation.

Tip: Drugs with greater potency are not necessarily more effective than drugs with less potency, and the drugs that are more effective due to their potency may not be the correct choice. You would not select the more potent drug for a client who complains of slight pain or give a less potent drug for severe pain. You are responsible and accountable for making critical clinical judgments in these situations, and choices must be based on evidence-based practice.

Curious factors can affect the action

Continuing on with our movie example and the study of drug action, we must consider factors that affect action. In a movie, the director, the actors, the lights, the props, and the extras all influence how the movie flows. A major factor that facilitates the flow of drug action and response is the dose of drug, or the amount of the drug given. Some drugs stimulate an immediate effect, such as epinephrine, which may be given when a person has an anaphylactic response to a foreign substance. For example, if a client who is allergic to bee stings is stung. Most drugs, however, do not demonstrate an immediate effect until a blood level is attained.

The type or classification of drug must be noted in a drug reference or database because all drugs are not equal and are used for different reasons. More than one drug may be given to treat a specific condition for an additive effect. Two drug classifications may be administered together for an added benefit—for example, furosemide (diuretic) and atenolol (beta-blocker) to reduce a client's blood pressure when the client has hypertension.

The route of administration has a great effect upon the action of the drug and the resulting responses. The time and frequency at which the drug is administered must be considered to maintain blood levels for therapeutic effects and avoid adverse reactions. Some drugs are given only once, and others are given every few hours at scheduled times with specific dosages to obtain the desired effect.

Despite caregivers' best intentions, sometimes a client will develop either a hypersensitivity to a drug or a full-blown anaphylactic reaction, which is life threatening. When either of these occurs, the client has had prior exposure to the drug or a component of the drug and has developed antibodies. A hypersensitivity reaction is a type of allergic reaction and is an "immune-mediated response to a drug agent in a sensitized client" (Reidl and Casillus 2003). A client can become hypersensitive or allergic to a drug at any time. Because hypersensitivity and allergic responses are unpredictable and unrelated to dose, beware and observe all clients for signs and symptoms of a drug reaction. Symptoms vary, but may include a rash, fever, itching, nausea, vomiting, and diarrhea. More serious symptoms may exhibit in the client including anxiety, restlessness, facial swelling, a thick tongue (caused by edema), difficulty breathing, and cardiovascular collapse. These serious symptoms require emergency treatment.

Watch out: Psychological factors also must be considered. When medications are administered to upset or anxious clients, the drugs may not be as effective. The setting is also important to consider. When given sedation, a client in a relaxed environment will be more responsive than if the drug is administered to a client in an environment with a lot of motion and confusion.

Thinking about action

Drugs can impact other drugs, with the combination causing an increased effect compared to when the drugs are given individually. One drug intensifies the potential of the other, causing an increased drug response from the combined effect, known as potentiation.

Similar to the action of potentiation is synergism: when two drugs that have similar actions are taken together and cause a more intensified response than if either drug is taken alone. When taken separately, drugs are not usually hazardous, but the combined effect can cause serious harm. An example of synergy would be combining alcohol with tranquilizers. The combination may activate a response in the brain that could result in coma or death. On occasion, some drugs cause a response that is unexpected or totally the opposite of what is desired. This type of undesired effect is referred to as an idiosyncratic reaction. An example would be when a sedative is given to cause sedation and calm in a client, and the opposite effect of excitement and agitation occurs.

Are you looking for a fight?

Throughout our movie, there is always a chance that the actors will experience a dramatic conflict with one another. Altercations can occur at any time due to miscommunication or daily annoyances that stimulate a roar between members of the cast.

Similarly, when drugs are administered, a reaction that is hypersensitive or allergic can arise without notice at any time, even if the client has taken the particular drug in the past. This type of reaction is unpredictable and unrelated to the amount of drug given. Some hypersensitive reactions to drugs can even occur one to two weeks after the drug was initially administered. Serum sickness demonstrates this type of reaction. It is normally treated by discontinuing the drug, administering antihistamines, and corticosteroids. The degree of response also varies from mild with a rash to full-blown anaphylactic shock during which a life-threatening response characterized by respiratory distress and circulatory collapse may occur. In this case, emergency treatment is required immediately.

Ask: Do you feel comfortable with your knowledge of anaphylactic drug reactions? Would you be able to distinguish the difference between a hypersensitivity response and a full-blown anaphylactic reaction? Do you know what to do? Take a moment to quiz yourself by jotting down characteristics of each.

Click: Some Internet resources for anaphylactic reactions include the following

www.anaphylacticreactions.com
www.aaaai.org/ar/
www.emedicine.com/EMERG/topic25.htm

The danger of sequels: Building up a tolerance

When a client becomes tolerant of a drug, it means that it takes more of the drug to obtain an effect because the body has become physiologically adjusted to the drug. The client must take a larger dose to produce a similar effect. If one Tylenol with codeine tablet used to get rid of a migraine headache, but now it takes three or more to be pain-free, this may indicate that the client has become tolerant to the drug or that something else is wrong. The client runs the risk of overdose by taking more than the prescribed dose to treat his or her headache. Often, the healthcare provider will change the drug rather than continue to increase the dose to avoid problems with drug tolerance and toxicity.

Cross-tolerance occurs when another drug of a similar classification is taken and larger doses are needed to produce the intended effect. When tolerance or cross-tolerance occurs, it is usually related to a change in the activation of drug metabolizing enzymes within the liver, which causes an increase in drug metabolism and excretion. Another reason for drugs failing to elicit the same effect as when the client initially took them is the decreased numbers and sensitivity of receptor sites.

"If you can't describe what you are doing as a process, you don't know what you are doing."

—W. Edwards Deming

Chapter 4

The route can change the story

The route through which a drug is administered is essential to consider. Often, the healthcare provider will write an order with several routes for you to consider. When preparing to administer a drug to the client, you must select the route based on the order and the client's current status. For example, healthcare providers often write for acetaminophen, "PO or PR for fever." The effectiveness, potency, time it takes for a drug to begin to work, and the reason why the drug is being given must be reviewed.

During an emergency, when rapid absorption is needed, an intravenous (IV) blood pressure drug such as Hyperstat may be administered IVP (IV push) for a hypertensive crisis. The effect is immediate. Another example is when albuterol, a bronchodilator, is given via nebulizer to treat a client having an asthma attack. Again, the action begins as soon as the drug enters the bloodstream to relieve the client's bronchoconstriction and facilitate breathing. In contrast, hydrocortisone ointment administered topically for a skin rash would be effective over a period of time through repeated applications. Be discerning when considering the route of drug administration if given that responsibility.

Open audition: Types of drug routes

ROUTE	ABBREVIATION	EXAMPLE	INSTRUCTIONS
By Mouth	PO	325 mg aspirin PO qd	Take tablet, capsule, or liquid by mouth according to directions on bottle.
Sublingual	SL, sl	gr 1/150 nitroglycerin SL PRN angina	Place tablet or liquid under tongue.
Inhalation	IH	2 puffs of albuterol b.i.d. MDI (metered dose inhaler)	Insert drug canister into plastic holder. Shake well; spray to test. Instruct client to breathe out through mouth expelling air and hold lips tight around mouthpiece. While inhaling, spray drug by pushing down on top of MDI. Hold breath. If another dose is required wait, one to two minutes, then repeat. Cleanse mouthpiece after using.
Intravenous	IV	Keflex (cephalexin) 1 gram (1000 mg) IV q8h	Administer via IV secondary line (piggyback) often via infusion pump.
Intramuscular	IM	Demerol (meperidine) 50 mg IM q4h PRN pain	Select site—deltoid, thigh, ventrogluteal, dorsogluteal—aspirate, if no blood flashback noted, then administer (45 to 90 degree angle to site) intramuscularly. Document site.
Subcutaneous	SQ, SC, Subq	Regular Humulin Insulin 10 units SQ q AM	Administer to subcutaneous site. Rotate site to prevent lipodystrophy. Document site.
Intradermal	ID	IPPD (1 dose 0.5 mL) intradermally (ID)	Administer at 30 degree under dermis to make wheal. Document site.
Intrathecal		Ziconotide 0.1 mcg (micrograms) intrathecally per hour via IV infusion	Administered by physician or advanced practice nurse.
Transdermally		Nitroglycerin patch 0.4 mg q12h	Make sure the area is clean. Remove transparent cover on patch and do not touch inside of patch. Apply patch to appropriate area.

Open audition: Types of drug routes (cont.)

ROUTE	ABBREVIATION	EXAMPLE	INSTRUCTIONS
Nasal spray and drops		2 gtts neosynephrine each nare b.i.d. for congestion	Instruct client to sit with head tilted backward for drops, or slightly forward accordingly if spray. Apply drops or spray. Inhale, repeat with other nostril as directed. Keep head in tilted back position for about 5 minutes for drop absorption. Do not blow nose immediately after administration. Clean dropper or sprayer.
Eye drops and ointments	OD (right eye) OS (left eye) OU (Both eyes)	Apply 1 gtt of gentamycin opthalmic drops to both eyes b.i.d.	Instruct client to tilt head backward and look up away from dropper or applicator. Pull down lower lid of designated eye. Place one drop into lower conjunctival sac, not directly onto cornea. Press gently upon the medial nasolacrimal canthus (close to nose) with tissue to avoid systemic absorption. Ask client to blink several times and then keep eyes closed for a few minutes. For ointment, pull down lower lid to view conjunctival sac of designated eye, squeeze a line of ointment onto the conjunctival sac. *Do not place directly on cornea.* Repeat for other eye as directed. Ask client to keep eye(s) closed for several minutes. Vision may appear blurry temporarily.
Ear drops	AD (right ear) AS (left ear) AU (Both ears)	Apply 2 gtts of otic cortisporin both ears b.i.d.	For children, administer by straightening the external ear canal by pulling down on the auricle. For adults, administer by pulling up and back on the auricle. Instill prescribed number of drops and ask client to remain in position with head

Open audition: Types of drug routes (cont.)

ROUTE	ABBREVIATION	EXAMPLE	INSTRUCTIONS
			tilted toward unaffected side for several minutes to prevent drug from being expelled out of the ear.
Pharyngeal		Cepacol spray for sore throat PRN.	Ask client to open mouth (tongue blade may be used) and spray toward back of throat.
Skin		Hyrdrocortisone ointment one application to affected area b.i.d	Apply thin layer of ointment to affected area.
Rectal	PR, pr, per rectum	One glycerin suppository PR q.d.	Have client lie on left side (Sim's position). Use gloves, lubricate suppository, then insert.
Vaginal	Vag	Administer one application of monistat cream b.i.d. vaginally	Apply with lubricated applicator to client in lithotomy position.

Steer clear of these villainous routes

You must be mindful and give medication by the correct route. For example, if you have an order for Keflex, don't inadvertently give the medication intended for the IV route through the gastrointestinal tube. Be sure to know the route of administration. The following table presents more examples of incorrect routes and some suggestions to prevent these errors.

Avoid villainous routes

Incorrect route	Suggestions to prevent errors	Read equipment labels
Oral medications given intravenously	✓ Note the prescribed route from original physician's order. Make sure the route is appropriate. ✓ Never give oral medications via IV, ✓ Be familiar with unit dose syringes, containers, and packaging for oral medications- ✓ Verify route prior to administration.	Medicine cups for oral medications. *Note:* Oral syringes for *oral use only.*
Enteral medications given parenterally	✓ Note the prescribed route from original physician's order. Make sure the route is appropriate. ✓ Verify tubing and bags for type. IV bags and tubing are not the same nor interchangeable. ✓ Verify that equipment is placed in appropriate pump.	• Read labels! (Enteral feeding tubing reads for enteral feedings and IV tubing reads for IV tubing.) • Enteral feeding pumps and IV infusion pumps *are not interchangeable.*
Intramuscular medications administered intravenously	✓ Note the prescribed route from original physician's order. Make sure the route is appropriate. ✓ Verify safe dose and route of parenteral medication. ✓ Ask when unsure about route of parenteral medication.	• Read physician orders carefully • Be familiar with usual routes for medications and verify each order individually.
Epidural and intravenous line confusion	✓ Note the prescribed route from original physician's order.	• Assess lines and tubing and connections from infusion to client. Label to avoid confusion.

Avoid villainous routes (cont.)

Incorrect route	Suggestions to prevent errors	Read equipment labels
	Make sure the route is appropriate. ✓ Label each line. ✓ Label each pump. ✓ Verify any time pump is adjusted and follow line by holding in hand until connecting point. ✓ Verify route prior to administration.	
Using IV syringes to measure oral doses of medications	✓ Note the prescribed route from original physician's order. Make sure the route is appropriate. ✓ Verify route prior to administration.	• Oral syringes are for oral medications and are not sterile. • Syringes for injections/drawing up IV medications are distinguished by syringe luer lock tip and are sterile.
Using intravenous medications orally	✓ Note the prescribed route from original physician's order. Make sure the route is appropriate. ✓ Examine labels from the pharmacy; they will often say: *FOR ORAL USE ONLY.* ✓ Verify route prior to administration.	Read labels. The pharmacy will send unit doses marked for Oral Use or for Injection Only at most institutions. Always verify!

Script questions

The following questions may assist in developing a priority list for choosing an appropriate route for drug administration:

✓ What is the drug prescribed for?

✓ Why is the patient receiving the drug?

✓ Has the patient been interviewed for any drug allergies?

✓ Is immediate drug action necessary, or is the drug being used to achieve an effect over time?

✓ Did you determine the prescribed route?

✓ Is there more than one possible route to select from to achieve the desired effect?

✓ Review the dose, frequency, and form of the drug to be administered.

✓ What is the onset, peak, and duration for the drug according to the prescribed route?

✓ When can the drug be expected to take effect?

✓ Is this the first time the client has taken the prescribed drug or has the drug been taken before with a known response?

✓ Always assess for potential adverse reactions.

✓ Document the patient's response to the drug: Was the intended effect achieved? Were any side effects noted?

 Fact: "Treatment of drug-related injuries adds at least $3.5 billion annually to the nation's healthcare bill, not counting indirect costs such as lost income and ancillary health and home care services," according to members of the IOM [Institute of Medicine] Committee on Identifying and Preventing Medication Errors, in a report called *Preventing Medication Errors*. (Osterweil 2006)

Intravenous drug administration is a familiar plotline

Administration of drugs via IV is one of the most commonly used routes, and it can be either the most beneficial or detrimental routes for clients. Just like the actors in our hypothetical movie, each player is assigned a specific role. You have a precise role regarding the administration of medications.

This role includes assessing the client prior to administering any drug to ensure client safety and interviewing the client for any allergies or past reactions to the prescribed drug.

Additionally, in the case of IV drug administration, you would consider the following checkpoints prior to implementing any IV drug:

✓ Is the client's IV site patent?

✓ Are there any signs of inflammation or infiltration?

✓ Is there a maintenance IV fluid?

✓ Is the infusion intermittent?

✓ What type of IV fluid is being used?

✓ Is the IV fluid compatible with the IV drug?

✓ Is the IV drug compatible with the IV additives (e.g., 20 mEq of potassium)?

✓ Are there any other IV solutions running through a "Y" set and, if so, are they compatible with the IV drugs to be administered?

✓ Over what period of time is the drug stable once activated or mixed, as in the case of add-a-bag where the drug is in the vial attached to a small volume of IV fluid and is activated by twisting and pushing the stopper to activate the device?

PG: Provider guidance for the elderly

 Watch out: The top 10 dangerous drug interactions in long-term care

Warfarin (coumadin) + NSAIDs*
Warfarin (coumadin) + Sulfa drugs
Warfarin (coumadin) + Macrolides
Warfarin (coumadin) + Quinolones**
Warfarin (coumadin) + Phenytoin
ACE inhibitors + Potassium supplements
ACE inhibitors + Spironolactone
Digoxin (lanoxin) + Amiodarone
Digoxin (lanoxin) + Verapamil
Theophylline + Quinolones**

*NSAIDs class does not include COX-2 inhibitors
**Quinolones that interact include: ciprofloxacin, enoxacin, norfloxacin, and ofloxacin

"Knowledge is of no value unless you put it into practice."

—Anton Chekhov

Chapter 5

Preparation makes the forum

Just like actors in a movie cannot be too prepared to deliver an award-winning performance, you can never be too prepared to administer drugs. Take a moment to compile an inventory regarding how to prepare to administer drugs wisely, safely, and through evidence-based research. Think about the following:

- What would you do first?

- How would you prioritize your actions?

- When obstacles occur, how would you demonstrate prudent critical thinking?

- Are you the type of person who is tempted to cut corners to save time/energy?

- Will cutting corners make your drug administration as safe or less safe?

Physician's orders, the reason why the client is receiving the drug, the prescribed route, the frequency of administration, assessment parameters, expected responses, special drug monitoring, and blood levels all must be considered each time you administer a drug to a client. In addition, you must seek additional clarification from healthcare providers/pharmacists if any questions arise to be sure everything is correct before giving the drug.

Watch out: A nurse enters a client's room to administer drugs. She has checked them against the medication record for the correct dose and time. She addresses the client by name and then proceeds to verify the client's identification band. The client then asks the nurse, "What is the little red pill for?" The nurse hesitates for a moment and then replies nervously, "The doctor ordered this medication for you."

Think about where the nurse has fallen short in her preparation. It is clear that she is lacking in either removing the packaging without reviewing it or not being able to identify the pill the client is speaking about. The nurse has not properly researched the drug before administering it. She was not able to demonstrate her preparation by offering the client an informed response as to what the drug was. Clients will often ask the nurse, "Why am I getting this drug?" or, "What is this medication for?" It is the nurse's responsibility as a licensed professional to perform the proper drug research and be prepared to administer drugs. Any other scenario is just plain unsafe. **As the nurse, you are accountable for correct preparation for drug administration.**

The six rights of administration make their debut

When preparing to administer any drug to a client, consider what is referred to as the "Five Rights" of medication administration:

✓ Right client

✓ Right route

✓ Right drug

✓ Right dose

✓ Right time

A *sixth right* often mentioned, but not a part of the original five rights, is the right documentation.

 Don't forget: Administer the drug to the client first, and then document. Documenting beforehand is considered falsification of documentation and is a violation of the nurse practice act.

 Tip: Developing good habits when it comes to delivering care to clients, including drug administration, is the key to being prepared. Here are some crucial factors that will assist you in being prepared:

✓**Time management** Generally, the time for medication administration lends to some flexibility, within reason. Most agencies allow for administration of drugs from 30 minutes before to 30 minutes after every hour. For instance, if a medication is scheduled for 0800, you could administer the medication from 0730–0830. The exception to this is for drugs such as chemotherapy, which have to be given exactly on time, or you run the risk of interrupting the chemotherapy protocol. Also, administering IV medications first affords the opportunity to administer other medications or care activities while the infusion is running.

✓**Organization** You must be organized. Each nurse has his or her own style of discerning how to accomplish nursing activities in an orderly fashion. Many nurses organize their medications and care activities using a worksheet. This way, each nurse has a blueprint of the care activities and time frame within which he or she can accomplish the assigned tasks.

✓**Priority setting** Setting priorities is essential in the healthcare environment. You must learn to set priorities around drug administration and other care activities. Moreover, you must be flexible, because often within a single day, priorities will have to be reordered due to changes in client conditions and physician orders.

✓**Evaluation** Continuously evaluate your performance in terms of delivering care and achieving ordered care activities. There always seems to be more to do than it seems reasonable to accomplish, and often you may feel challenged to get everything done. Performing self-evaluation can assist with being more effective. Asking questions such as, "How could I have prioritized more effectively in this situation?" or "How could I have improved my time management?" may prove helpful. Based on this evaluation, you can assume a new plan of action for the future.

"*You must be the change you want to see in the world.*"

—Mahatma Gandhi

Considerations and cautions to keep in mind as the director

Route of Administration	Forms	Considerations	Caution
PO (by mouth) or GI tube	Tablets	May contain dyes, preservatives, and other inert additives. Dissolves in gastric fluids. Administer with 8 oz of water to facilitate dissolution.	Some clients are allergic to the dyes and inert additives.
	Chewable	Appealing flavors, colorful. Often in children's form.	Keep all medications away from children to avoid accidental overdose. Flavorful medicines are attractive to children. Do not refer to medications as candy.
	Enteric Coated	Dissolves in small intestine instead of stomach. Advantage: used for drugs that normally cause gastric irritation.	DO NOT CRUSH or CHEW. Crushing or chewing removes protective coating which protects gastric lumen from irritation.
	Extended release (XL) Sustained release (SL) Long acting (LA)	Prolonged action, timed release and slow action 12-24 hours duration. Contain large amount of active drug. Come in various	NEVER CRUSH or GIVE ORALLY! Crushing and given by mouth or through a GI tube administers a bolus of drug; overdose can be toxic leading to death!
	Capsules	sizes, some are gelatin and others are solid, referred to as caplets. Administer with 8 oz of water to facilitate dissolution.	May contain fillers and preservatives.
	Extended release (XL) Sustained release (SL)	Prolonged action, timed release, and slow action	NEVER SEPARATE CAPSULE OR ADMINISTER BEADS orally or through a GI tube, as bolus of

Considerations and cautions to keep in mind as the director (cont.)

Route of Administration	Forms	Considerations	Caution
	Long acting (LA)	12-24 hours duration. Contain large amount of active drug.	drug constitutes overdose and may be lethal! Instruct clients not to bite, chew, or separate capsules.
	Solutions	Absorb more rapidly because they do not need to be dissolved.	Measurement is extremely important. Use appropriate measuring devices.
	Suspensions	Shake well. Suspensions can separate with medication collecting on towards lower half of container.	Unshaken and unmixed suspensions deliver the wrong concentration of medication even if measured correctly!
	Throat Lozenges	May contain sugar. May change the taste of food and beverages temporarily.	Clients should be cautioned not to fall asleep with lozenge in mouth, as it's a choking hazard. Not appropriate for very young children.
	Pharyngeal Sprays	Aim spray toward back of pharynx. May alter the taste of food temporarily.	
Sublingual (SL)		Placed under the tongue. Dissolves quickly. Taste may be unpleasant.	Store in original containers to prevent decomposition.
Buccal		Between cheek and gum. Immediate dissolution. Taste may be unpleasant. Medication absorbed rapidly into bloodstream.	Client should rinse mouth to avoid mucosal irritation.
Parenteral (IV, IM, SQ, ID)	Solutions	IV immediate action SQ Immunizations, Insulin, Heparin	Use sterile equipment. Do not confuse oral syringes with parenteral syringes.

Considerations and cautions to keep in mind as the director (cont.)

Route of Administration	Forms	Considerations	Caution
		IM Immunizations, pain medication ID Tuberculin Skin Test Allergen testing.	Use appropriate size needles. Measure exact amounts to ensure correct dosage. Aspirate for IM injections to prevent systemic administration. Give clear instructions to client regarding follow-up for tuberculin skin test reading and allergen testing.
	Suspensions		Use larger bore needles since suspensions are thick.
Topical to Skin	Creams	Apply to affected area.	ADMINISTER AS PRESCRIBED. Caution clients to follow instructions exactly. Applying additional doses of steroid creams will cause changes in integrity of the skin such as atrophy.
	Lotions	Apply to affected area.	Administer as prescribed. Shake lotions prepared by the pharmacy well to prevent separation of ingredients.
	Ointments	Apply to affected area.	Administer as prescribed.
Inhalation (Nasal inhalation, metered dose Inhalation (MDIs)	Solutions/Sprays	MDI canisters must be shaken so drug will be mixed within container. Instruct clients to test spray first before administration.	Instruct clients to wash mouthpiece of metered dose inhaler (MDI) after each use, especially with inhaled steroids. Failure to do so can cause candidiasis of the mouth and other infections. Use as directed; overuse can cause respiratory distress. Store as directed.
	Powders	Measured dose per inhalation	
Eye	Solutions	Moisturizers for eye. Used for eye infections. Used for eye analgesia from trauma.	Keep sterile. Administer as directed. Can be systemically absorbed and cause adverse reactions.

Considerations and cautions to keep in mind as the director (cont.)

Route of Administration	Forms	Considerations	Caution
	Ointments	Moisturizers for eye. Used for eye infections.	Keep applicator sterile. Administer as directed.
Ear	Solutions	Used for ear infections.	Keep applicator sterile. Administer as directed.
Vaginal	Creams	Commonly used to treat vaginal infections.	Variable absorption.
	Suppositories	Commonly used to treat vaginal infections.	Variable absorption.
Rectal	Creams	Steroid based creams. Creams to reduce hemorrhoidal edema.	Variable absorption.
	Ointments	Steroid based ointments. Ointments used to reduce hemorrhoidal edema.	Instruct clients to administer as directed. Variable absorption.
	Suppositories	Laxatives, analgesics, sedatives, antipyretics.	Variable absorption.
	Solutions	Enemas. Used for bowel evacuation.	Overuse can cause fluid and electrolyte imbalances.

Chapter 6

The plot thickens: Therapy and adverse reactions

Drug therapy is the science of using drugs to treat illness, cure disease, and manage an array of symptoms from a multitude of conditions. It ranges from the most basic, such as taking an aspirin for minor arthritis pains, to treating complex conditions, such as cancer and AIDS. Put simply, without access to drug therapy, the quality of our lives in terms of morbidity and mortality would be very different. In countries where drug therapy is not accessible or even available, quality of life and longevity is greatly affected. In the healthcare delivery system, prescribing and administering drugs is an essential part of the treatment plan.

Decisions regarding the type of drug, route, frequency, and expected outcomes are made by the expert healthcare professional based on evidence in practice. Drug therapy is not a precise science, but it is based on assessment, implementation, evaluation, and research. Therapeutic outcomes vary dependent upon genetics, ethnicity, weight, age, diet, external environment, other drugs in the body, physical and emotional condition, and an individual's response to a particular drug.

Earlier in this section, we discussed pharmacokinetics (the movement of drugs throughout the body) and pharmacodynamics (the action of drugs upon the body in terms of absorption, metabolism, distribution, and elimination). We explored the impact the various routes of drug administration can have upon the body.

As a nurse, you must consider throughout your own research how drugs affect the body and be cognizant of the fact that individuals may react differently to the same drug. For example, due to reduced kidney and liver function the elderly and children may metabolize the same drug differently than a young or middle adult. The elderly metabolize and excrete drugs more slowly due to their age, while young children metabolize and excrete drugs less effectively due to immature organs and their inability to handle large doses of drugs. Metabolic rates are higher in children; therefore, doses are calculated based on body weight. Children should never be considered small adults. Oftentimes, dosages for drugs used for similar reasons will have to be adjusted for age and size.

Carefully . . . finding . . . the . . . steady . . . state

It is common practice for drugs to be administered in repeated doses so a steady state can be achieved. A steady state is the amount of drug administered equal to that of the amount being metabolized or excreted. Some drugs require careful monitoring of plasma levels due to difficulties in obtaining and maintaining a steady state of equilibrium. In such cases, blood levels may be drawn to achieve drug ranges within what is referred to as a therapeutic window or therapeutic index. The therapeutic window (index) is considered the concentration above which the drug is toxic and below which the drug is ineffective. This therapeutic range is usually small, and increments in between are significant. There is little difference between toxic and therapeutic dosages, so monitoring of blood levels of the drug is critical. The peak level of a drug is the highest therapeutic blood level, and the trough is the lowest blood concentration level. Peak levels are drawn 30 minutes to two hours after the drug is administered, depending upon the route. Trough levels are obtained approximately 30 minutes prior to the next scheduled dose.

For example, when gentamycin, an IV antibiotic, is prescribed, therapeutic blood levels are monitored and peak and trough levels obtained. The trough level would be drawn 30 minutes before the next scheduled dose and the peak would be obtained one hour after the IV administration was completed.

 Ask: What are the drugs that require peak and trough level monitoring? Take a moment to jot down a few.

Beware the villain that is adverse drug reactions

According to the Food and Drug Administration (FDA) Center for Drug Evaluation and Research (CDER), two-thirds of client visits result in a prescription, and adverse drug reactions (ADR) increase exponentially with four or more medications. More than 2 million serious ADRs occur yearly resulting in more than 100,000 deaths. ADRs are the fourth leading cause of death, ahead of pulmonary disease, diabetes, AIDS, pneumonia, accidents, and automobile deaths. (CDER 2002).

Serious ADRs are defined by the FDA as events caused by a drug that result in a patient's death, hospitalization, disability, cause a congenital abnormality, life-threatening event, or require an intervention to prevent permanent damage. ADRs are common, significantly contribute to morbidity and healthcare costs, and carry the single greatest risk for harm to patients in hospitals. It has been estimated that more than 770,000 people per year who are hospitalized in the United States suffer ADRs, which costs major hospitals up to $5.6 million per year. This estimate does not include ADRs resulting in admissions, malpractice, and litigation costs, or the costs of injuries to patients. National hospital expenses to treat patients who suffer ADRs during hospitalization are estimated to be between $1.56 billion and $5.6 billion annually (Ostenberg and Blaschke 2006).

With this information in mind, be aware that any drug can cause an ADR in the client. Therefore, when healthcare providers prescribe drugs to treat illnesses, manage symptoms, and cure diseases, they weigh risks versus benefits of the drugs that are prescribed. *There is no completely safe drug.* All drugs have potential adverse effects upon the human body.

Side effects: The unfriendly sidekicks

The terms adverse reactions and side effects are often used interchangeably in the literature. Some literature correctly refers to adverse effects or ADRs as more serious events than expected side effects for drugs. For example, metronidazole (Flagyl) is a drug that is used to treat infections. A side effect of metronidazole is metallic taste. This side effect may be annoying for a brief time, but it is not life threatening. The drug causes a metallic taste in the mouth either by changing the chemical composition of the saliva or by temporarily affecting the taste sensors in the mouth. Conversely, some drugs such as indomethacin (Indocin), a potent nonsteroidal anti-inflammatory drug (NSAID), can cause a rare, but serious life-threatening adverse effect called agranulocytosis, which is a severe and dangerous reduction of white blood cells.

The key to reducing ADRs is through awareness and recognition of potential problems. Drug errors are usually due to human error—regardless of whether harm results in the client. Common causes of errors include

- look-alike or sound-alike medications

- illegible handwriting

- misinterpreted or misplaced decimal points

- wrong drug, wrong client, wrong time, or wrong dose

You can prevent ADRs by following the practices validated by evidence-based research and using discerning clinical skill when administering drugs.

Tip: Avoid potential serious ADRs by

- performing drug research prior to the administration of any drug

- practicing the basic "Five Rights" of drug administration: *right client, right drug, right dose, right route, right time*

- Assess the client at frequent intervals, especially when a drug is initially administered

- Alert the physician immediately upon noticing any signs and symptoms of potential problems

- Document actions taken to manage adverse events

- Educate the client about signs and symptoms so they can report any potential problems to healthcare providers

"Whenever you are asked if you can do a job, tell 'em, 'Certainly I can!' Then get busy and find out how to do it."

—Theodore Roosevelt

Chapter 7

Take 5, people: A quick word about dosage calculations

Returning again to our movie example, drug calculations are like an actor's lines in the movie, and an actor must know his or her lines very well—just like you, as a nurse, must know your drug calculations very well.

One pitfall that nurses encounter is forgetting dosage calculation formulas. Repeatedly reciting their lines ensures that the actors won't forget them and will deliver a grand performance. Likewise, repeatedly practicing dosage calculations will ensure that you understand how to do them and continue safe practice with drug administration. Memorizing the formulas is key to correct calculation of drug dosages. You have a legal obligation to know how to calculate drug dosages, so there is no room for guesstimating.

Keep a good clinical calculation book handy for any review you deem necessary and quiz yourself periodically to stay fresh. Even though you may not have had to do a manual calculation in a while, you are always accountable for being able to do it correctly. The alternative could be detrimental for your client. Review the basic drug calculation formulas on the next page.

> "Do what you can, with what you have, where you are."
>
> —Theodore Roosevelt

Basic calculation formulas

D =   desired dose (of the drug ordered by the physician)

H =   on-hand dose (of the drug dose on the label of the bottle, vial, ampule, etc.)

V =   vehicle (form or amount in which the drug comes—tablet, capsule, liquid, suspension, etc.)

X =   unknown (the number of tablets, capsules, or mL to administer)

Dose divided by on-hand amount times vehicle method

D/H x V = X (amount to give)

Or

Ratio: Proportion

Known		::		Desired	
H	: V	::	D	:	X
On hand	Vehicle		Desired dose	Amount to give	

Example: The physician orders Keflex capsules 500 mg PO q.i.d.

On hand: cephalexin capsules 500 mg

How many capsules should the nurse administer for the correct dose?

2000/500 X 1 capsule = 4 capsules

or

500 mg : 1 capsule :: 2000 mg: X capsule(s)

500X = 2000

X = 4 capsules

IV flow rate formula for continuous infusion

Amount of fluid ÷ hours to administer = mL/hr

Example: The physician orders 1 liter of D5 1/2NS with 20 mEq KCL/ L to be administered over eight hours. For how many mL/hr should the nurse program the IV pump?

$$1000 \text{ mL}/8 \text{ hours} = 125 \text{ mL/hr}$$

IV flow rate for intermittent infusion (secondary set or piggyback)

$$\frac{\text{Amount of solution x gtt/mL (set)}}{\text{Minutes to administer}} = \text{gtt/ min}$$

Example: The physician orders 500 mL over 4 hours. The nurse has an IV set with a 10 gtts/mL factor. For how many gtts/min will the nurse adjust flow regulator?

$$\frac{500 \text{ X } 10}{4 \text{ (60 min)}} = 20.83 \text{ repeating} = 21 \text{ gtts/min}$$

IV flow rate for intermittent pump

$$\text{Amount of solution} \div \frac{\text{minutes to administer}}{60 \text{ min/hr}}$$

Math rule: $\dfrac{\text{Amount of solution x } 60 \text{ min/hr}}{\text{Minutes to administer}} = \text{mL/hr}$

Example: The physician orders Unasyn 2 grams IV q 8 hours. The nurse has on hand a secondary bag of Unasyn 2 g in 100 mL of NS. The nurse will administer the infusion over 20 minutes. For how many mL/hr will the nurse program the IV infusion pump?

$$100 \text{ mL} \div 60 \text{ mL}/20 \text{ minutes}$$

$$100 \text{ mL x } 20/60$$

$$1{,}200/60 = 33.3 \text{ mL/hr}$$

Eyes forward and you may begin

Try a few practice problems:

1. The physician orders erythromycin 250 mg PO q.i.d. Available are

erythromycin 250 mg tablets. How many mg should the nurse administer per day?

2. The physician orders a heparin drip at 950 units per hour. Available is heparin 25,000 units in 500 mL of 0.9 % NACL. For how many mL/hr should the nurse program the IV infusion pump?

3. The order reads morphine sulfate 3 mg IV now. Available is morphine sulfate 4 mg/2 mL. How many mL should the nurse administer?

4. The client is receiving cefalzolin (Kelfex) 2 g IV q 8 hours. The client weighs 110 lbs. The safe dose in the drug book is 50 mg/kg/day. What is the top safe dose? Is this client receiving a safe dose?

5. The physician orders methylprednisolone (Solumedrol) 40 mg IV. Available is methylprednisolone 40 mg in 100 mL of D5W. The nurse determines that the medication should infuse over at least 45 minutes. For how many mL per hour will the nurse program the infusion pump?

6. The physician orders 1 liter IV maintenance fluids D5 1/4 NS with 20 meq KCL/L over 10 hours. For how many mL/hr will the nurse program the IV infusion pump?

Answers:

- 1000 mg per day

- 19 mL/hr

- 1.5 mL

- 2,500 mg top safe dose, yes

- 75 mL

- 100 mL/hr

Fact: There are risks with any drug. Acetaminophen can cause liver damage, NSAIDs can cause gastrointestinal bleeding, and aminoglycosides can cause kidney damage.

Chapter 8

No stunt men needed: It's better to be safe than sorry

It's better to be safe than sorry—famous last words, but so true. The actors in a movie would not dare show up to the set unprepared. If they did, they would most likely lose their part to another actor. Each day that a nurse clocks into work, it is a new day, and preparation takes center stage. Every day is one filled with possibility and challenge, a day filled with concentration and exhaustion. But even so, you, as a nurse, have the responsibility to the client to give an outstanding performance filled with safe, effective care based on knowledge and critical thought. Clients' lives are in the hands of the nurses and doctors caring for them.

There are times when nurses do not put their best foot forward, when drugs are not properly researched, and attempts are made to cut corners in drug administration. When a client asks the nurse about his or her drugs and the nurse clearly doesn't know the answer, the client loses faith in the nurse—not only in his or her ability to administer medications, but in all areas.

An Oscar-worthy acronym

You must practice safety through SAFE: *Safe Administration* of drugs through *Foundation* of knowledge and *Evaluation*:

S — Safety first! You must be safe in practice.

A — Administration of drugs is predominantly your responsibility. You must be prepared to administer drugs to clients.

F — Foundation of knowledge is required for practice in terms of the principles of drug administration, action, and awareness of adverse reactions.

E — Evaluation must be done on a continuous basis by the nurse incorporating life-long learning and ongoing research.

This acronym should serve as a reminder for vigilant practice.

"Life is inherently risky. There is only one big risk you should avoid at all costs, and that is the risk of doing nothing."

—Denis Waitley

Part Two

Okay, now it's time to delve a little deeper. Let's head into the actor's studio with drug interactions and explore topics such as compatibility, food and drink, nutrients, and herbs. We are well on our way to creating an engaging, thought-provoking story about safe practice.

Chapter 9

Setting the stage with a good foundation

The foundation for a good movie, along with having a good story, is having talented actors. You need actors who research their character, come prepared to the set, and have a willingness to work. You also need a creative director, a producer, and a crew who collaborate to pull everything together.

So what does having a good foundation mean in terms of nursing and drug administration?

Understanding drug interactions is about having a good knowledge foundation and being aware that the foundation is not static—it's always expanding. A critical knowledge foundation has many attributes and is related to an individual's professional discipline. For example, a lawyer has a very specific knowledge base that is different from that of a nurse or a physician. A nursing foundation of knowledge is very diverse. You must be knowledgeable in many areas and be able to put that knowledge into action at a moment's notice.

 Don't forget: Drug manufacturers present detailed information regarding drug preparation, such as amount and type of fluid to dilute with PO, IM, and IV drugs. It is crucial for you to take note of this information, because not preparing a correct dilution can alter the drug's effectiveness or result in injury to the client.

Thrown into the spotlight

You begin building your foundation for nursing practice by attending nursing school and then passing the NCLEX® licensure examination. But learning and growing in experience and expertise by no means ceases upon graduation and licensure. The true tests of character, clinical and communication skills, and critical thought and perseverance happen when a person enters the profession.

With drug administration, you must be knowledgeable, safe, skillful, and able to communicate with the client in a partnership with the healthcare team. The goal is to assist the client and to improve his or her health/comfort. Through diligence, you will continue to research drugs (yes, this means looking up every drug that you are not familiar with every time). There will always be many convenient resources available, and a short amount of time invested will benefit the client beyond measure.

 Fact: You must recognize that drug administration requires life-long learning and continued research.

> *"Good judgment comes from experience,*
> *and experience comes from bad judgment."*
>
> —Barry LePatner

Chapter 10

A behind-the-scenes look at drug interactions

Adverse drug reactions (ADR) and drug interactions affect many clients' lives each year with unexpected illnesses, hospitalization, and even death. A number of deaths each year are attributed to clients taking new prescription drugs and combining them with existing medications. Also, a small number of drugs are withdrawn each year from the market and labeled as harmful or lethal due to increased client mortality or morbidity.

There is a growing consciousness about drugs among consumers, with more and more people becoming aware of their need to be educated about all the drugs that they take. With this in mind, as a nurse, you have an obligation and responsibility to check for drug combination safety when administering drugs to clients.

A drug interaction is a chemical reaction that occurs when one drug is altered by pharmacological effects of another drug, food, or substance given concurrently. The end result may be either exaggerated or diminished effects of one or both drugs. Other times, a new effect emerges that is not observed with either drug alone.

Drug interactions are becoming more prevalent, especially since clients obtain prescriptions from more than one healthcare provider. Additionally, over-the-counter (OTC) medications, vitamins, and supplements all contribute to an alarming polypharmacy—taking a combination of drugs for various ailments. These drug interactions alter effects on drug action by either an increase or decrease of available drug, inhibition or initiation of metabolism between drugs, minerals, vitamins, dietary supplements, and other chemical exposures within the environment.

Monitoring the action among the drug players

Several mechanisms serve as the catalyst for drugs interacting with drugs, food, and other substances. These mechanisms include the absorption, distribution, metabolism, and elimination of a drug within the body.

Changes in absorption affect drug activity and action. Drugs are absorbed into the bloodstream and then travel to their site of action. Diminished absorption occurs as a result of alteration of blood flow to the intestine, alteration of the drug in the intestine, increased or decreased gastric motility, alterations in stomach acidity, and changes in the bacteria within the intestine. Also, be aware that drug absorption can be affected by a drug's ability to dissolve, the impact of changes caused by other drugs, and food and substances that bind to the drug.

Drugs administered directly via IV or IV push (IVP) cause immediate drug action because the process of absorption does not occur. As soon as the drug enters the bloodstream, its effects are activated. Therefore, exercise extreme caution when giving drugs via the IV route and consider potential problems prior to administration.

Through the process of metabolism, drugs are converted into other substances such as metabolites in order for the body to eliminate through the kidneys. The majority of drugs are eliminated through the kidney—either unchanged or as a metabolite of the drug—by the liver. The liver and kidney are critical sites for potential drug interactions. Drug interactions can increase a desired effect or exaggerate an undesired effect of the drugs administered.

Drug interactions are complex because of their unpredictability. Factors essential to consider when trying to avoid drug interactions are prior interactions, age, lifestyle (diet and exercise), disease conditions, doses of drugs, physiology, and psychology of the client.

Some commonly used drugs are more likely to interact with other drugs when the client takes a combination of them. These drugs often combine with the other drugs to increase, decrease, or block effects. When you review a client drug list or the medication administration record, a red flag should promptly wave.

Watch out: Here are some examples of commonly used drugs that interact with other drugs:

- Anticoagulants and aspirin (↑ risk of bleeding)

- Antacids and anticoagulants (↓ absorption of anticoagulants)

- Antacids and beta-blockers (atenolol, propranolol ↓ effectiveness)

- Antacids and iron (↓ iron absorption)

- Acetaminophen and alcohol (↑ risk of liver damage or gastrointestinal bleeding)

- Antihistamines and other central nervous system depressants (antianxiety, antipsychotic, opioid, sedative-hypnotic drugs, monoamine oxidase inhibitors, and tricyclic antidepressants ↑ sedative effects that can lead to coma and death)

- Insulin and beta blockers, ace inhibitors, and other oral antidiabetic drugs (↑ effects)

- Iron and allopurinol (↑ iron in liver)

Whew! And these are just a sampling to whet your whistle! The list goes on—but . . .

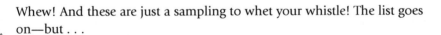

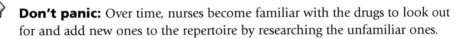

Don't panic: Over time, nurses become familiar with the drugs to look out for and add new ones to the repertoire by researching the unfamiliar ones.

Know your lines

You can reduce the number of potential drug interactions by taking the following actions:

- Ask the client if he or she is allergic to any medications or foods

- Assess the client prior to administering the medication

- Review the physician's orders prior to administering the medication

- Verify the physician's medication orders, and if they are unclear or do not make sense, contact physician for clarification

- Review generic and brand names of medications; there are many sound-a-like or look-a-like drugs

- Know reason why medication is being administered

- Check safe dose of medications prior to administration

- Be aware of onset, peak, and duration of medication

- Verify safety for all drug combinations by researching beforehand

- Be familiar with side effects/adverse reactions to watch for in client

- Determine whether the medication should be taken with or without food

- Consider food or other drug interactions when giving PO medications

- Know how long a parenteral drug is stable when reconstitution is necessary

- Know IV tubing "Y" set incompatibilities (incompatible drugs when administered together will develop crystals and or precipitate, which is extremely dangerous)

- Discern whether IV fluids are compatible with IV drugs

- Check expiration dates of all equipment, medications, and solutions

- If drugs appear to look different or funny, do not administer; verify with pharmacist that the drug looks the way it is supposed to as prepared

- Use the basic "Five Rights" of medication administration for every drug given

- Store medication correctly until it's is needed (whether medication has to be protected from light or refrigerated, etc.)

Fact: "Health professionals also use computer systems with drug-interaction screening software, electronic prescribing, and other technology," says Mark Langdorf MD, chair of the department of emergency medicine at the University of California, Irvine. "In a busy emergency room, you have to quickly find out what a patient is taking and how those drugs could interact with other treatments." (*www.fda.gov/fdac/features/2004/404_drug.html*)

A variety show of interactions

The actors in the movie must interact with each other so that the momentum of the action continues. Some of the interactions are desired, and other times, there are conflicts between the members of the cast. Interaction means activity between more than one person, place, or thing. With drugs, an interaction occurs when two chemicals influence or change each other.

In Chapter 3, we discussed specific types of drug interactions including agonist, additive, potentiation, synergism, antagonist, idiosyncratic, hypersensitivity, and allergic responses. In addition to these, there are specific drug-to-drug, drug-to-food or -beverage, and drug-to-dietary supplement interactions. A drug-to-drug interaction occurs when drug action is changed in a manner in which the effects manifested would not occur otherwise if the drug were administered alone. The combination of two or more drugs has the potential to cause a reaction that is desired, undesired, or has unpredictable effects. For example, antacids should not be administered concomitantly with tetracycline antibiotics because the two drugs interact with one another where the antacid decreases the effects of the antibiotic.

Another example of a more serious interaction is with IV phenytoin (Dilantin) and IV fluids that contain dextrose. A dangerous reaction occurs when the phenytoin and dextrose mix. It is contraindicated for phenytoin and dextrose containing IV solutions to be used together.

Nurses who were not conscientious and did not check compatibility between other drugs and IV fluids prior to administration have found out the hard way that when phenytoin and dextrose are mixed in the same IV line, a crystalline precipitate forms immediately upon contact, which creates a frightening scenario for the nurse and the client.

 Watch out: How would the nurse know if the client was having an adverse drug reaction?

- A sudden change in a client's condition soon after drug administration

- Change in level of consciousness

- Dangerous drop in blood pressure

- Extremely elevated blood pressure

- Rapid irregular heart rate

- Abnormally low heart rate

- Change in respiratory rate with noticeable distress

- Fever

- Damage to vital organs such as the heart, liver, or kidneys

- Blood dyscrasias, aplastic anemia, agranulocytosis

- Pseudomembraneous colitis

- Superinfection

- Cardiovascular collapse

- Less severe symptoms may include rash, itching, nausea and vomiting, diarrhea, and headache

Click: Check up on your drugs!
www.drugdigest.org/DD/Interaction/ChooseDrugs/1,4109,,00.html
www.drugs.com/xq/cfm/pageID_1150/qx/index.htm
www.healthatoz.com/healthatoz/Atoz/drugdb/drugSearch.jsp

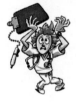

Don't panic: Some hospitals have Micromedex, a comprehensive database where nurses can look up evidence-based information on drugs, drug interactions, and client teaching. This service is often linked to systems on computers in the medication room and at bedside computers for easy accessibility.

"As a general rule, the most successful man in life is the man who has the best information."

—Benjamin Disraeli

Chapter 11

Welcome the special guest star, cytochrome P450

It is essential that you appreciate the potential of cytochrome P450 enzymes and its subfamily (CYP2D6, CYP1A2, and CYP3A4, etc.) to cause drug interactions. Cytochrome P450 enzymes are important because they assist in drug metabolism by inducing chemical reactions that reduce substances toward being more water-soluble so they can be excreted from the body via the kidneys. Cytochrome P450 enzymes generally function by two mechanisms: enzyme inhibition or enzyme induction.

Enzyme inhibition involves drugs competing for other enzyme binding sites and usually causes a decrease in drug efficacy. Enzyme induction is initiated when a drug activates the synthesis of more enzyme proteins, which facilitates the enzymes metabolizing ability. Enzyme inductors cause diminished drug effects in most cases. The induction or inhibiting effects that occur when a drug interferes with the cytochrome P450 pathways can cause serious physiological effects that may be potentially fatal.

The following are examples of the drug classifications to pay particular attention to:

- Antidepressants (especially selective serotonin reuptake inhibitors and tricyclics)

- Antianxiolytics

- Antipsychotics

- Antihistamines

- H2 receptor blockers (cimetidine)

- Beta-blockers

- Narcotics

- Theophylline

Specific drugs within the cytochrome P450 category and what specific drug combinations to avoid can be referenced in any good drug guide.

 Click: For further information regarding the cytochrome P450 enzyme system and drugs within specific categories:

www.anaesthetist.com/physiol/basics/metabol/cyp/Findex.htm#cyp.htm
http://medicine.iupui.edu/flockhart/
www.globalrph.com/cytochrome.htm

"It's a job that is never started that takes the longest to finish."

—J. R. R. Tolkien

Chapter 12

Beware of actors that lack compatibility

Incompatible drugs, when combined together, form alien compounds that are unpredictable and dangerous. Drugs may not be compatible with other drugs, IV fluids, in Y-site IV connections, and in the same syringe. You must consider the stability of the drug by itself and when combining it with another drug. Through reviewing evidence-based research of the drug, you can determine the safety of mixing it, drawing up more than one drug in the same syringe, connecting the IV drug at the Y-site, adding a medication to an IV solution, or running a subsequent IV solution with the drug. Drug compatibilities must be considered with all formulations, including tablets, liquids, solutions, injections, and topical applications. When exploring drug compatibilities, you may find that drug stability varies according to several factors.

Tip: Here are some factors that influence drug stability:

- Changes in pH

- Light can change the composition of the drug

- Temperature can change the composition of the drug

- Additives may influence the stability of a drug solution

Or indications that a change has occurred:

- Color changes indicate a chemical reaction has occurred and has changed the original drug form

- Odor may indicate that a chemical reaction has occurred

- Precipitate are solid particles formed from a chemical reaction

- Crystallization are crystals that form as the result of chemical reaction

Drug instability and incompatibility must be considered every time you administer a drug to a client. Drug incompatibilities are a real risk, as precipitates and crystals can form as the result of incompatible drug interactions and can clog IV lines or, more seriously, cause an embolus in the unsuspecting client.

SAS and SASHes—not just for costumes!

It is essential that you know the principles of IV therapy. One safety net to help with this is to practice the SAS and SASH techniques when administering IV medications, IVP medications, or IV intermittent/secondary/piggyback medications. First, here's **SAS**:

> **S**aline
> **A**dministration
> **S**aline

SAS is the practice of flushing the IV site or saline port connected to the client with saline, then administering the drug. When the drug has infused through the IV tubing or IV port, a saline flush is used again to clear any remaining drug in the IV tubing so the client receives all of the drug. This also prevents drug interactions when other drugs are administered through the same IV line the next time a medication is administered.

Now take a look at **SASH**:

> **S**aline
> **A**dministration
> **S**aline
> **H**eparin (Lock)

With SASH, a saline flush is administered. Then the drug is administered, and after the drug has infused, a saline flush is administered. Then, a very dilute heparin called HepLock is used to maintain patency (i.e., to keep the vein from clotting).

Make sure actors work nicely together

Clients who have debilitating conditions or are unable to eat are prescribed nutrition that is administered via IV through central venous access ports. Total parenteral nutrition (TPN) formulations must be checked for compatibility with drugs intended to be administered through IV Y-sites.

The following drugs are *not compatible* with TPN:

- Acyclovir, Adenosine, Albumin, Amphotericin, Ampicllin*, Ativan*, Atropine

- Dilantin

- Epinephrine

- Flurouracil*

- Ganciclovir sodium*

- Imipenem-cilastatin sodium

- Phenobarbital*

- Pipercillin sodium

- Rifampin

- Sodium bicarbonate

- Versed

- Zofran*

* dependent upon TPN formulation (check with drug resource)

 Watch out: IV Dilantin (phenytoin) must not be mixed with any other medications or IV solutions with Dextrose. A crystal precipitate will form immediately and present a danger to the client. Dilantin (phenytoin) is compatible with 0.9% NaCl.

 Ask: Be sure to interview your client, asking what medications have been taken, so you can avoid giving a drug that could be incompatible. Drugs administered by mouth can interact with other PO medications. Clients who have taken an incompatible combination may complain of nausea and vomiting, abdominal pain, or dizziness.

 Click: For more information:
www.arrowintl.com/documents/pdf/education/ml-ng1201.pdf

> *"One important key to success is self-confidence. An important key to self-confidence is preparation."*
>
> —Arthur Ashe

Chapter 13

Drugs with a supporting cast of nutrients

Like the scenes that make up our movie, nutrients such as vitamins and minerals are essential building blocks. Nutrients promote the healthy functioning of all the systems within the body. Deficiencies of vital nutrients and minerals can lead to malnutrition, chronic conditions, and be the precursors to many diseases. Thus, as a nurse, you must consider the scheduling of medications that could potentially cause drug-nutrient interactions at times relative to meals.

Healthcare providers include an assessment regarding the client's nutrition and make recommendations within the plan of care. For example, orthopedic clients who have undergone bone surgery are likely to have vitamins ordered on the medication list, such as vitamin C, D, E, calcium, and zinc, to promote optimal healing and bone regeneration. Another example is antacids, which are commonly administered in hospitals, doctors' offices, and nursing homes to elderly clients who may also suffer from anemia and have iron preparations prescribed. Teach clients not to take antacids and iron concomitantly, because when they are given at the same time, the result is decreased iron absorption.

You can become more familiar with the influence that diet has on drug administration through assessment of clients and continued research. Becoming familiar with common drug and nutrient interactions is the first step toward becoming more attune to potential medical concerns with the client.

Drug-nutrient reactions get mixed reviews

CLASSIFICATION	EXAMPLE OF DRUG	INTERACTION WITH NUTRIENT
Alcohol	Ethanol	↓ absorption of fat, retinol, thiamin, cobalamin and folate; alteration of storage and utilization of retinol; ↑ urinary excretion of zinc and magnesium
Analgesics/NSAID	Aspirin	↑ urinary excretion of ascorbic acid (vitamin C); potential for gastrointestinal bleeding and subsequent iron deficiency; ↑ folate and vitamin D requirements
Antacids	Aluminum or calcium containing	↓ iron, copper, phosphate, and magnesium absorption
Antibiotics	Penicillins Aminoglycosides Chloramphenicol	↑ urinary excretion of amino acids; ↓ intestinal vitamin K and cobalamin synthesis, potential malabsorption of fat, cobalamin, calcium, magnesium, and carotenoids
Anticoagulants	Coumadin	Vitamin K ↓ and tocopherol ↑ drug effect
Anticonvulsants	Phenobarbital Phenytoin	Folate antagonists; ↑ vitamin D, vitamin K, and pyridoxine requirements; ↓ vitamin D metabolism leading to hypomagnesemia, hypocalcemia, and hypophosphatemia
Antidepressants	Imipramine	May cause riboflavin deficiency; ↑ appetite
Antihypertensives	Hydralazine	Pyridoxine antagonist; ↑ urinary excretion of manganese and pyridoxine
Antimalarials	Pyrimethamine Sulfadoxine	Folate antagonists
Antineoplastics	Methotrexate	Folate anagonist; may cause impairments of fat, calcium, cobalamin, lactose, folate, and carotene absorption
Antitubercular	Isoniazid	↑ metabolism of pyridoxine—subsequent pyridoxine deficiency blocks conversion of

Drug-nutrient reactions get mixed reviews (cont.)

CLASSIFICATION	EXAMPLE OF DRUG	INTERACTION WITH NUTRIENT
		tryptophan to niacin leading to niacin deficiency; ↓ calcium absorption; ↓ conversion of vitamin D by the liver
Antiulcer	Cimetidine	↑ cobalamin absorption
Cardiac Glycosides	Digoxin	↑ urinary excretion of calcium, magnesium, and zinc; Anorexia.
Corticosteroids	Hydrocortisone Prednisone Dexamethasone	↓ calcium and phosphorus absorption; ↑ urinary calcium, potassium, ascorbic acid, zinc, and nitrogen excretion; ↑ pyridoxine and vitamin D metabolic requirements
Diuretics	Furosemide Thiazides Spironolactone	↑ urinary potassium, sodium, chloride, magnesium, zinc, and iodine excretion; ↓ calcium excretion leading to hypercalcemia and hypophosphatemia with thiazides, ↑ calcium excretion with furosemide; ↑ urinary sodium and chloride; ↓ urinary potassium excretion
Hypocholesterolemic Agents	Cholestyramine Colestipol	↓ absorption of fat, fat soluble vitamins, calcium, cobalamin, folate
Laxatives	Bisacodyl Phenolthalein Mineral Oil	Abuse leads to general malabsorption, steatorrhea, and dehydration; ↓ absorption of fat soluble vitamins, electrolytes, calcium
Oral Contraceptives		↑ folic acid, and possibly pyridoxine and ascorbic acid requirements; ↓ calcium excretion, impaired tryptophan metabolism
Stimulants	Caffeine	↑ urinary calcium excretion

Adapted with permission from The University of Washington Medical Center (http://healthlinks.washington.edu/nutrition/section8.html.)

Click: Some additional resources on drugs and nutrients:
www.ext.colostate.edu/PUBS/foodnut/09361.html
http://clinicalcenter.nih.gov/ccc/patient_education/drug_nutrient

Please your audience

Remember these tips for avoiding drug-nutrient interactions to help keep clients safe:

- Verify physician orders

- Check common nutrient interactions against current medication list

- Research drug-nutrient interactions with drug references or facility-approved online resources (e.g., Micromedex)

- Determine whether drug should be administered on an empty stomach or with food or water

- Administer vitamin and mineral supplements before or after other medications

> *"It's not enough that we do our best; sometimes we have to do what's required."*
>
> —Sir Winston Churchill

Chapter 14

Snack time: Drug-food interactions

Because eating food is a normal activity of daily living, it may be difficult to think that the food most of us savor each day could be detrimental to our health or even lethal when combined with drugs. The presence of food in the gastrointestinal (GI) tract can interact with a drug by

- facilitating absorption

- impairing absorption

- slowing GI motility

- changing GI pH

- interfering with GI enzymes

- exhibiting a chemical reaction with immediate physiological responses ensuing within the body

A potentially life-threatening food-drug interaction occurs when a monoamine oxidase inhibitor (MAOI), a type of antidepressant, is taken with foods high in tyramine, a potent vasoconstrictor. When a food high in tyramine is ingested with a MAOI antidepressant drug, a severe hypertensive crisis or hemorrhage within the brain can result. Healthcare providers prescribe

MAOIs last when treating depression, because clients must adhere to a strict diet free from any tyramine-laden foods.

Watch out: Clients taking MAOI antidepressants must be counseled to prevent severe or fatal adverse events. The following is a list of foods high in tyramine and therefore must be *avoided*:

- Ale (beer)

- Avocados

- Bananas

- Beans (lima beans, butter beans, bean pods)

- Caviar

- Chocolate

- Cheese (especially aged cheeses)

- Coffee

- Figs

- Fish (smoked or pickled herring)

- Liver (beef or chicken)

- Processed meats (bologna, fermented meat, salami, pepperoni, summer sausage)

- Raisins

- Raspberries

- Sour cream

- Soybeans or sauce

- Tofu

- Wines (especially red)

- Yeast

- Yogurt

In addition, clients taking lithium, an antidepressant, should avoid eating any foods with excessive salt, which can decrease drug effects. At the same time, too little salt in their daily diets can lead to increased serum lithium levels. Another example of a food-drug interaction is when clients take ace inhibitor drugs with potassium-rich foods, which can result in hyperkalemia. Furthermore, absorption and effectiveness are reduced when dairy products are combined with tetracycline and fluoroquinolone antibiotics.

There is much to consider when combining food and drugs. Client education is essential to ensure safety and proper administration of medications to avoid severe reactions.

Enjoy a coffee break . . . or maybe not

Beverages can also be associated with drug interactions. Alcoholic beverages, beverages with caffeine (e.g., soda, chocolate, energy drinks, coffee, and tea), dairy or calcium-fortified beverages, and citrus juices can all have an effect when administering drugs.

Grapefruit juice interacts with a long list of drugs, causing increases in drug effectiveness that can prove toxic or even lethal. Anticoagulants interact with many foods and drugs, which either cause greater efficacy, increasing the client's potential for hemorrhage, or render the drug ineffective, placing the client at risk for developing life-threatening blood clots. The antibiotic metronidazole (Flagyl), when combined with alcohol, causes a severe reaction that may include flushing, tachycardia, palpitations, nausea, and vomiting.

Caffeine is a type of drug in and of itself, a xanthine derivative similar to the respiratory drug theophylline, which can result in physiologic effects including central nervous system stimulation, increased heart rate, blood pressure, hyperglycemia, cerebrovascular vasoconstriction, increased secretion of gastrointestinal acids, skeletal muscle stimulation, and bronchodilation.

Caffeine is an additive in other pharmaceutical preparations: OTC analgesics (Excedrin, Anacin) and prescription medications such as (Cafergot), which is used to treat migraine headaches.

Alcohol metabolizes much like drugs do. It is a central nervous system depressant. Alcohol and alcohol-containing products (e.g., cough syrup preparations) cause drug interactions from mild to severe depending upon the drug and the amount of alcohol ingested.

Alcohol intensifies many drugs that affect the central nervous system, and when combined with antidepressants, antipsychotics, antianxiety medications, narcotic analgesics, hypnotics and sedatives, or anticoagulants, can cause severe consequences.

Be careful when casting these characters: Common food-drug interactions

There are specific drugs within classifications commonly known to cause food-drug interactions of which you should be particularly aware. All other drugs should be checked for potential reactions prior to administration to the client.

When dealing with food, be wary of these commonly known drug classifications:

- Alcohol
  - Ace Inhibitors
    - Anticancer drugs
      - Anticoagulants
        - Antihypertensives
          - Antiseizure drugs
            - Benzodiazepines
              - Calcium channel blockers
                - Fluoroquinolones
                  - HIV-1 protease inhibitors
                    - Lithium
                      - NSAIDs
                        - Monoamine oxidase inhibitors
                          - Statins
                            - Tetracyclines
                              - Tricyclic antidepressants

Watch out: The following table lists foods that are high in vitamin K and therefore reduce the effectiveness of coumadin (Warfarin):

Foods high in Vitamin K	
Alfalfa sprouts	Dried beans
Avocado	Green leafy vegetables
Broccoli	Green tea
Brussels sprouts	Kale
Beef	Liver
Cabbage	Oats
Cauliflower	Onions, green scallion
Collard greens	Soy products
Escarole	Watercress

Click: For more information on coumadin, click here:
http://ods.od.nih.gov/factsheets/cc/coumadin1.pdf
www.ptinr.com/data/pages/section.aspx?z=13&l=fb

Prop class: Insight into enteral feedings

Dilantin (phenytoin), warfarin (coumadin), and the fluoroquinolone antibiotics (ciprofloxacin, levofloxacin, ofloxacin, moxifloxacin, and gatifloxacin) are frequently prescribed and are well-known to interact with many enteral feedings. Bioavailability is affected where drugs bind to the protein in the feeding formula, resulting in less free drug availability. Coumadin (warfarin) may interact with enteral feeding formulas that contain vitamin K in the solutions. For this reason the following recommendations are made:

- *For fluoroquinolone antibiotics,* hold enteral feedings for one to two hours before and one to two hours after administration

- *For phentoin* (Dilantin), hold enteral feedings for one to two hours before and one to two hours after the dose is administered

- *For coumadin* (warfarin), hold enteral feedings one to two hours prior to the dose and one to two hours post dose administration

Click: Look up the following for food-drug interactions:
http://cpref.gsm.com/inter.asp?r=8084
> a. aspirin
> b. ciprofloxacin
> c. phenelzine
> d. felodipine

Click: For more information on food-drug interactions:
www.druginteractioncenter.org/
www.fpnotebook.com/ID145.htm
www.nclnet.org/Food%20&%20Drug.pdf
www.globalrph.com/drugfoodrxn.htm

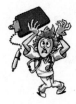

Don't panic: Remember, in order to administer drugs safely, there are many things that you must consider to avoid food interactions. Again, don't panic! Databases and references are available for quick research so nurses can perform drug administration activities in a timely manner.

> "Habit is habit and not to be flung out of the window by any man, but coaxed downstairs a step at a time."
>
> —Mark Twain

Chapter 15

An herb documentary: Is green always keen?

Sometimes green does not mean go. Green, simply put, is not always keen.

Herbs have been touted as natural products that can heal the mind, body, and spirit. They have been categorized as supplements and are easily found next to the vitamins at your favorite grocery or corner drug store. Products considered natural remedies for ailments may be in fact hazardous to your health—when combined with other over-the-counter or prescription drugs, herbs can cause liver or kidney damage, or, worse, cause death.

For centuries, natural cures have been passed along as folk remedies that people swear by: vinegar, honey, and water as a natural treatment for arthritis; chamomile tea deemed to calm frazzled nerves; and bee pollen for energy. Although some natural products may be safe enough and some individuals may experience real benefits from them, many herbal treatments have not been proven to be safe—taking them is at one's own risk.

Self-treatment for aches, pains, and common maladies may not be a wise choice. Herbs are drugs that are not regulated by the Food and Drug Administration. Their authenticity and potency are not verifiable. Specialists can be sought who can make recommendations and prescriptions regarding herbal products used for medicinal purposes. Naturopathic physicians and pharmacists with training in homeopathy pharmaceuticals are the professionals to contact to obtain advice about natural remedies. Physicians and pharmacists should coordinate with traditional healthcare providers when the client seeks medical attention from multiple providers.

Too much advice can confuse an actor

When our actors seek recommendations for improving their performance from the director, producer, other actors, friends, and family, the mix of suggestions may get confusing regarding who said what, when, and what to do. Similarly, when clients have multiple healthcare providers and obtain prescriptions for medications while also shopping the health food store to stock up on herbal preparations, the client may unknowingly be setting up for many confusing symptoms and interactions between drugs and natural products. This is an untold, unsafe situation.

Recently, providers within the healthcare system have taken notice of the problem with clients self-medicating with natural products, which, in turn, create lurking dangers unbeknownst to them. As part of health assessments, healthcare providers should interview clients about the medications they currently take and inquire as to whether they take any herbs or supplements.

 Tip: Routinely ask the client whether he or she takes any herbs, or diet or vitamin supplements. Obtaining this information when taking history assessments can ward against potential adverse situations when other drugs are prescribed or the client undergoes any type of surgical intervention.

Carefully choose your supporting cast

Herb	Classification	Therapeutic Use	Drug Interaction
Arnica	Anti-infective	Insect bites, bruises, acne, boils, sprains, muscle, and joint pain.	Alcohol (↓ efficacy); antihypertensives (↓ efficacy); anticoagulants (↑ efficacy); antiplatelet agents (↑ risk of bleeding).
Chondroitin	Non-opioid analgesic	To relieve symptoms of joint pain.	Anticoagulants (↑ risk of bleeding); antiplatelet agents (↑ risk of bleeding); cephalosporins (↑ risk of bleeding); NSAIDs (↑ risk of bleeding); thrombolytics (↑ risk of bleeding).
Dong Quai	None	Blood purifier, menstrual cramps, irregularity, and menopausal symptoms. Vasodilating and antispasmodic effects.	Alcohol (↑ risk of bleeding); anticoagulants (↑ risk of bleeding); antiplatelet agents (↑ risk of bleeding); cepalosporins (↑ risk of bleeding); NSAIDs (↑ risk of bleeding); valproates (↑ risk of bleeding).
Echinacea	Anti-infective, Antipyretic	Bacterial and viral infections, prophylaxis and treatment of upper respiratory illnesses (cough, colds), wounds and burns, urinary tract and yeast infections.	Immunosuppressant interactions due to the herbs. Also has immunostimulant activity. May interact with anabolic steroids, antifungals [{ketoconazole}↑ efficacy]; methotrexate (↑ efficacy); midazolam (↑ efficacy).
Garlic	Lipid lowering agent	Prophylaxis for cardiovascular disease, prevention of colorectal and gastric disease.	Anticoagulants (↑ risk of bleeding); antiplatelet agents (↑ risk of bleeding); contraceptive drugs

Carefully choose your supporting cast (cont.)

Herb	Classification	Therapeutic Use	Drug Interaction
			($\downarrow$ efficacy); cyclosporine ($\downarrow$ efficacy); protease inhibitors ($\downarrow$ plasma concentrations); thrombolytics ($\uparrow$ risk of bleeding).
Ginger	Antiemetic	Relief of nausea and vomiting from chemotherapy, motion sickness. May be used for dyspepsia, flatulence. Decreases cholesterol.	Anticoagulants ($\uparrow$ risk of bleeding); antidiabetic agents ($\uparrow$ hypoglycemia); antiplatelet agents ($\uparrow$ risk of bleeding); calcium channel blockers ($\uparrow$ hypotension); thrombolytics ($\uparrow$ risk of bleeding).
Ginkgo Biloba	Antiplatelet agent, Central Nervous System Stimulant	Use for short term memory deficit, inability to concentrate, depression, improves peripheral circulation, sexual dysfunction.	Aniticoagulants ($\uparrow$ efficacy); antiplatelet agents ($\uparrow$ efficacy); cephalosporins ($\uparrow$ risk of bleeding); insulin (altered dose requirement); MAOIs ($\uparrow$ efficacy); NSAIDs ($\uparrow$ risk of bleeding); thrombolytics ($\uparrow$ risk of bleeding); valproic acid ($\uparrow$ risk of bleeding).
Ginseng	None	$\uparrow$ energy to treat fatigue, antidepressant, sedative, immune response, and $\uparrow$ appetite.	Anticoagulants ($\downarrow$ efficacy); insulin ($\downarrow$ efficacy); oral hypoglycemics ($\downarrow$ efficacy); MAOIs ($\downarrow$ efficacy). May interfere with immunosuppressant therapy.
Glucosamine	Antirheumatic	Arthritis, glaucoma.	Antidiabetic agents ($\downarrow$ efficacy). May cause resistance to chemotherapy.
Kava Kava	Antianxiety agent, Sedative/hypnotic.	Anxiety, benzodiazepine withdrawal, insomnia, myalgia,	Benzodiazepines ($\uparrow$ efficacy); CNS depressants ($\uparrow$ efficacy);

Carefully choose your supporting cast (cont.)

Herb	Classification	Therapeutic Use	Drug Interaction
		menstrual cramps, PMS, stress.	levodopa (↓ efficacy); opioid analgesics (↑ efficacy). Use with DHEA, Coenzyme Q-10, and Niacin (↑ hepatotoxicity).
St. John's Wort	Antidepressant	Mild to moderate depression, topical ↓ inflammation, skin, wounds, and burns.	Alcohol (↑ CNS adverse reaction); antidepressants (↑ CNS adverse reactions); digoxin (↓ efficacy); MAOIs (↑ CNS depression and serotonin syndrome); SSRIs (↑ serotonin syndrome).
Valerian	Antianxiety, Sedative/hypnotic	Anxiety, insomnia.	Alcohol (↑ CNS depression); antihistamines (↑ CNS depression); CNS depressants (↑ efficacy); sedative/hypnotics (↑ efficacy).

Click: For more information about herbs and drug interactions, visit the following Web sites:

www.nlm.nih.gov/medlineplus/druginfo/herb_All.html

www.rxfiles.ca/acrobat/cht-herbal-di.pdf

www.ena.org/education/GENE/HerbsandDrugsInteractionhandout.pdf

> *"An investment in knowledge always pays the best interest."*
>
> —Benjamin Franklin

Chapter 16

Over-the-counter drugs: Too many actors can be confusing

In an age where there is a preoccupation with beauty, fitness, health, and nutrition, media of all types—newspapers, magazines, books, the Internet, and television—entertain flamboyant advertisements about "miracle pills" for optimal health, longevity, weight loss, and cures for diseases. There are even infomercials promoting both prescription and nonprescription over-the-counter drugs (OTC).

One might feel deprived if the medicine cabinet is not chock full of "just in case" prescriptions and OTC products. The gamut is broad, ranging from acetaminophen for headaches to laxatives for constipation.

OTC drugs do not require a prescription and are not regulated in the same way that prescriptions are. They are accessible by anyone at any corner grocery or drug store.

Polypharmacy creates a crowded stage

One term commonly referred to when speaking about drugs is polypharmacy. Polypharmacy denotes taking a combination of many medications for various ailments in the guise of being helpful (healthful) but can suddenly become a downward spiral of events. It's like having too many actors in a movie. Quickly, the audience can become confused, and a movie that was flowing along well becomes unwatchable.

It is the responsibility of healthcare providers to review individual drug lists with clients and try to economize the numerous prescriptions and OTCs being taken together. As a nurse, you can assist clients through counseling and education about drugs and their uses to avoid polypharmacy. Encouraging clients to keep their healthcare providers up to date on their medication lists (prescription and OTC) will circumvent more serious health concerns in the future.

OTC drugs can ruin a performance

There are many potential hazards with OTC drugs. Taking more than the amount recommended on a bottle of acetaminophen can cause liver damage, or worse, death. A common drug used for indigestion belongs to the family of cytocrome P450 (discussed earlier in chapter 11)—a potential danger lurking when clients obtain cimetidine (Tagamet) at their favorite grocery store. This drug interacts with a long list of other drugs.

Encourage clients to read drug labels and follow checklists for remembering good practices when taking drugs. The Food and Drug Administration recommends that the public read drug facts before taking any medications, as a precaution. Listed are the active ingredients, purpose of the drug, uses, warnings, side effects, pregnant and breast-feeding recommendations, directions for use, storage information, and a list of inactive ingredients.

See the next page for an example.

Drug Facts

Active ingredient (in each tablet)   **Purpose**
Chlorpheniramine maleate 2 mg.......................Antihistamine

Uses temporarily relieves these symptoms due to hay fever or other upper respiratory allergies:
- sneezing • runny nose • itchy, watery eyes • itchy throat

Warnings
Ask a doctor before use if you have
- glaucoma • a breathing problem such as emphysema or chronic bronchitis
- trouble urinating due to an enlarged prostate gland

Ask a doctor or pharmacist before use if you are taking tranquilizers or sedatives

When using this product
- you may get drowsy   • avoid alcoholic drinks
- alcohol, sedatives, and tranquilizers may increase drowsiness
- be careful when driving a motor vehicle or operating machinery
- excitability may occur, especially in children

If pregnant or breast-feeding, ask a healthcare professional before use

Keep out of reach of children. In case of overdose, get medical help or contact a Poison Control Center right away.

Directions	
adults and children 12 years and over	take 2 tablets every 4 to 6 hours; not more than 12 tablets in 24 hours
children 6 years to under 12 years	take 1 tablet every 4 to 6 hours; not more than 6 tablets in 24 hours
children under 6 years	ask a doctor

Other information store at 20-25° C (68-77° F)
- protect from excessive moisture

Inactive ingredients D&C yellow no. 10, lactose, magnesium stearate, microcrystalline cellulose, pregelatinized starch

Click: For further information regarding OTCs, check out these Web sites:
www.fda.gov/cder/consumerinfo/OTClabel.htm
www.fda.gov/womens/getthefacts/otc.html
www.fda.gov/womens/getthefacts/usemeds.html
http://familydoctor.org/852.xml

Be a hero and follow these recommendations

You can assist clients in the prevention of OTC interactions with other drugs by making the following recommendations:

- The client should know why he or she is taking the drug

- Encourage the client to read drug labels

- Advise the client to take only recommended doses as directed

- The client should talk to his or her healthcare provider or pharmacist before combining an OTC medicine with other OTCs or prescription drugs

- Review with clients how much of the drug to take, how often, how soon results can be expected, possible side effects, more serious adverse effects to watch for, and how long the medication should be taken

- Remember that you may be the healthcare provider that takes the extra time needed to fully prepare the client to take medications safely

> *"The best preparation for good work tomorrow*
> *is to do good work today."*
>
> —Elbert Hubbard

Part Three

What's a great movie without a memorable ending? It's time to look at drug interactions in seniors and children, and spend some time learning about evidence-based practice. Remember, combining all this knowledge will encourage audiences to give rave reviews when you are performing your drug interactions.

Chapter 17

Great communication leads to hit movies and healthy interactions

Communication is essential when interacting with other people. In our movie, the actors must communicate with producers, directors, other actors, and the crew. Without communication, the scenario would be disorganized chaos, and the movie would never materialize. But even with communication, maintaining a schedule and getting everything organized on the set can be extremely overwhelming.

In the healthcare environment, communication is the key that keeps a complex system functioning. Every person needs some type of healthcare service during their lifetime. The relationships and communication that emerge between clients and healthcare providers is paramount for both parties. Clients must be open in relaying healthcare information for correct diagnosis and treatment. Healthcare providers must develop a rapport with clients to obtain the necessary information for health histories and accurate assessments.

Filling all the roles

The plot thickens when considering a healthcare system that continues to hold the responsibilities of managing the care of multitudes of people 24/7 in a competent and accurate manner. There has been a strain on the healthcare system to keep up with the growing healthcare needs of the population, and that demand often exceeds resources. In an attempt to meet the needs of every individual, institutions have demanded more from healthcare professionals and staff just to complete daily tasks.

The end . . . for pen and paper

Most hospitals have some form of computer-assisted charting. In the past, nurses encountered dilemmas in trying to balance time consuming data entry and client care. Today, medications, labs, diagnostic tests, client information, and electronic Kardexes can all be managed from a computer. The days of pen and paper are gone. As a nurse, you will continue to be challenged to manage daily computer applications and provide hands-on care for clients.

Overloads have caused a river of errors for many in medication administration. In an attempt to reduce the number of adverse drug events, information systems were reviewed to establish protocols to deal with the problem. Computerized physician order entry (CPOE) emerged out of the need to reduce medication errors. The use of the computerized ordering for medications assisted with the reduction of medication errors by physicians, but it did not solve the problem on the administration level for clients.

Scanning is becoming a main character

In February 2004, the Food and Drug Administration (FDA) issued a final ruling that barcodes must be placed on most prescription and OTC drugs in an effort to enhance client safety and reduce medication errors. The FDA estimates that the barcoding method, once implemented, will result in more than 500,000 fewer adverse effects over the next 20 years. The implementation of the barcode method will assist in eliminating former medication errors such as

- wrong patient

- wrong dose

- wrong drug

- wrong time

- changes in the prescribed medication

Many healthcare institutions are in the process of updating their medication delivery systems to include barcoding. Nurses like you now have the added challenge of becoming familiar with the new technology and learning new equipment and protocols for medication administration. CPOE, barcoding, and electronic charting are here to stay. Individuals are the directors of this computer-assisted information age and are accountable for correct data entry. Despite the high-tech advancements, healthcare providers are obligated to maintain a balance between data entry and client care.

Click: For more information on barcoding, check out these Web sites:

www.fda.gov/oc/initiatives/barcode-sadr/fs-barcode.html

www.uspharmacist.com/oldformat.asp?url=newlook/files/Prod/oct00barcode.cfm&pub_id=8&article_id=607

> *"When people talk, listen completely. Most people never listen."*
>
> —Ernest Hemingway

Chapter 18

Take extra care
when working
with children

With infants and children at a high risk for prescription errors, administration errors, and serious drug interactions, it's important to take necessary precautions. Over the past 10 years, the Food and Drug Administration (FDA) reports, attention has been given to study pharmacological products in children. Two legislative initiatives emerged out of the concern to address pharmacological product development:

- The Best Pharmaceuticals for Children Act (BPCA), which studied drugs

- The Pediatric Research Equity Act (PREA), which focused on both drugs and biologicals

Historically, drug development in children has not been based on the same rigors of evidence as adults. But children and the elderly are more vulnerable to drug events, including route of administration mistakes, dosage miscues (including frequency), and narrow therapeutic indexes.

Some of the gaps that the FDA has identified include unnecessary exposure to ineffective therapies in the pediatric population, along with ineffective dosing and overdosing of effective drugs, which has significant effects on metabolism and drug clearance. As the result of discrepancies in appropriate prescribing practices and selection of products, pediatric adverse events have

increased. The new FDA labeling change—described in Chapter 22—addresses the pediatric labeling and prescribing recommendations in hopes of avert-
ing inappropriate prescribing practices and adverse drug events.

Kids are not stand-ins for adults

Tricycling in pediatrics is essential for the safety of our smallest clients.
Children are not little adults! The tricycle is the interdisciplinary approach
among physicians, nurses, and pharmacists in developing and maintaining
safe drug administration practices, from prescribing to drug preparation and
administration.

That said, what are some of the practices that you can implement to prevent
drug interactions in children?

- Prioritize drug safety interventions according to child's level of growth
  and development

- Always verify safe dosages

- Provide education to child/family

- Use accurate measuring devices such as oral syringes and medicine cups
  for exact amounts

- Check the color, shape, size, and smell of medicines

- Perform drug research regarding incompatible drugs

- Follow special instructions, such as taking the medication with or without food

Tips to talk to other directors

While you run the drug administration show for a child under your care, it's
necessary to pass the knowledge on to parents. After all, they'll be calling the
shots when they get home. Pass over the directorial duties to them with
these helpful tips:

Family education regarding safe administration of drugs for children

- Explain to parents that they should ask healthcare providers the name and reason for the medication
- Parents should know how much medication to give, how often, and how long the medication will be taken
- Encourage parents to ask what to do if the child misses a dose
- Support parents in obtaining any special considerations, such as how the medication should be taken with or without food
- To avoid overdose, do not crush pills unless given permission to do so
- Discuss common side effects
- Parents should demonstrate an understanding of when to stop the medication if adverse reactions arise and should be clear about parameters
- Call the healthcare provider/check with pharmacists about drug interactions, and taking supplements or herbs with the medication
- Teach children that medicines are not candy
- Describe how medication is stored at room temperature, in the refrigerator, or in containers that need to be protected from light
- Identify any potential hazards in the home to make medication administration child-safe
- Have poison control number (1-800-222-1222) accessible for instructions and call 911

Click: For more information on pediatric drug interactions and safety, check out these sites:

www.fda.gov/cder/pediatric/labelchange.htm
www.ahrq.gov/consumer/20tipkid.htm
http://aappolicy.aappublications.org/cgi/reprint/pediatrics;112/2/431.pdf
www.cdc.gov/ncipc/factsheets/poisonprevention.htm

> *"You can observe a lot just by watching."*
>
> —Yogi Berra

Chapter 19

Aging actors: Preventing drug misuse in seniors

The U.S. Census Bureau reports that beginning in 2011 the number of baby boomers aged 65 and over is projected to rise faster than the total population in all states. This population will continue to increase until 2030, when one U.S. citizen in five will be older than 65 years of age (Vestal 2005). The implications are enormous in terms of healthcare delivery and client education to ensure medication safety.

 Fact: According to the Department of Health and Human Services, almost half of Americans use at least one prescription drug. Prescription drug use is on the rise among people of all ages and increases as the population ages. Five out of six people 65 and older take at least one medication, with half the elderly taking three or more medications daily (HHS 2004).

Know when to say 'cut' when taking pills

Polypharmacy includes clients taking dosages that are too high, medications that are incorrectly prescribed or filled, and medications that interact with or duplicate the actions of other medications, herbal supplements, and OTC medications. There are conglomerations of possibilities that contribute to the concern about polypharmacy in the elderly population. In addition, some elders may become drug abusers—addicted to pain killers and other medications, replenishing their stashes by seeking services from multiple healthcare providers and pharmacies. Preventing adverse drug events can be a challenge with the building hazards unbeknownst to both the healthcare provider and client.

Symptoms of polypharmacy can be difficult to diagnose especially when the client has more than one healthcare provider prescribing drugs. Common complaints about symptoms that clients may make could be confused with the normal aging process, chronic disease, and side effects from medications.

Watch out: Common signs and symptoms easily confused with aging include the following:

- Constipation

- Diarrhea

- Incontinence

- Confusion and falls

- Tiredness, sleepiness, or decreased alertness

- Loss of appetite

- Depression or lack of interest in usual activities

- Weakness, dizziness, and tremors

- Visual or auditory hallucinations

- Anxiety or excitability

- Deceased sexual behavior

Remembering in black and white

Physiological changes that occur with the normal aging process contribute to the dilemma of polypharmacy and adverse drug events. Older livers and kidneys do not metabolize drugs as well as they did in the younger days. There is an increased risk for drug accumulation and toxicities, especially with drugs with narrow therapeutic indexes.

Many seniors take drugs to maintain normal body functioning, such as medications to lower blood pressure, maintain heart rates, maintain fluid balance, optimize gastrointestinal functioning, and manage musculoskeletal complaints such as arthritic pain. Patients taking pills to help manage each symptom and condition of aging can be challenging for healthcare providers. Compounded by the common complaints of aging such as decreases in mental acuity, balance, sensory acuity, mood and memory deficits, living alone and declining financial resources, healthcare providers face the task of treating without prescribing an overload of medications.

Another challenge remains to balance therapy with the elderly's ability to comply and follow directions correctly for their healthcare concerns. With the baby boomer population growing at an accelerated rate, medication errors continue to be of great concern for healthcare providers. The mere fact of the aging process predisposes older adults to adverse drug effects. Risk factors that complicate the care are polypharmacy, coexisting diseases, physiological changes, and the use of multiple healthcare providers. Nurses play a vital role in client education for the prevention of polypharmacy and adverse drug events.

 Click: The Joint Commission also pays great attention to improving the safety of using medication. Here's a look at the 2007 National Patient Safety Goals:
www.jointcommission.org/PatientSafety/NationalPatientSafetyGoals/07_npsg_facts.htm

Prevent catastrophic events

Here are some recommendations for prevention of polypharmacy and adverse drug events. These helpful tips can be passed along to seniors:

- Know the reason for your medications, how to take them, and for how long

- Maintain a current list of your drugs and take it with you to each doctor's appointment

- Keep a copy of your medication list with you at all times

- Ask your healthcare provider or pharmacist to use a database to check your drug list for drug interactions

- Make sure you understand how to take your medication correctly and whether there are any special instructions that require your attention

- Check with your healthcare provider about what action you should take if you miss a dose of your medication

- Check with your healthcare provider before using any over-the-counter (OTC) product or herbal supplement

- If you have problems with vision or memory, designate a family member or friend to assist with your medication administration

- Use a pillbox or calendar to assist you with remembering to take and organizing your medications

- When in doubt, ask your healthcare provider or pharmacist to review your medication list and instructions with you

- Be familiar with common side effects of the drugs you take

 Ask: And here are some tips for you. Ask these questions when assessing a client for polypharmacy:

- Do you take more than one prescription medication?

- Do you take any dietary supplements, vitamins, or OTC or herbal medicines?

- Do you have more than one healthcare provider providing you with prescriptions?

- Do you fill your prescriptions at more than one pharmacy?

- Do you live alone?

- Do you have problems with your vision or memory?

- Do you sometimes forget your medications?

- Do you have anyone to help you with your medications?

- What are your concerns regarding your medications?

 Click: For more information on polypharmacy in seniors, visit the following Web sites:

www.fda.gov/fdac/features/1997/697_old.html
www.cdc.gov/nchs/pressroom/04news/hus04.htm
www.nida.nih.gov/whatsnew/meetings/bbsr/prescription.html
http://jaapa.com/issues/j20050501/articles/polypharm0505.htm

> *"Choose the life that is most useful, and habit*
> *will make it the most agreeable."*
>
> —Sir Francis Bacon

Chapter 20

Dress rehearsal: Practice makes perfect

Actors in a movie practice their parts to be prepared for the performance. Nurses perform their parts in the healthcare arena each day by attending to the needs of clients. It is essential for nurses to develop exceptional practice habits. More important, nurses have an obligation to the client to implement care interventions based on research that is evidenced in practice. The days of performing care relying on "the way we have always done it" is no longer acceptable in an age of high stress, technological advancement, and litigation.

Developing expert practice habits will serve nurses well and protect clients from harm. **There are no acceptable excuses when it comes to client safety.** A different type of golden rule certainly applies: An ounce of prevention is worth its weight in gold.

What do nurses do in terms of practice? They are licensed healthcare professionals who are accountable for their individual practice. As a nurse, you have a responsibility for being familiar with the guidelines for nursing practice—called the *Nurse Practice Act*—for the state where you work. Specific guidelines are outlined in each state's nurse practice act regarding nurses' duties in regard to medication administration. There are standards of practice for medication administration that you are accountable for as designated by the State Board of Nursing to ensure public safety.

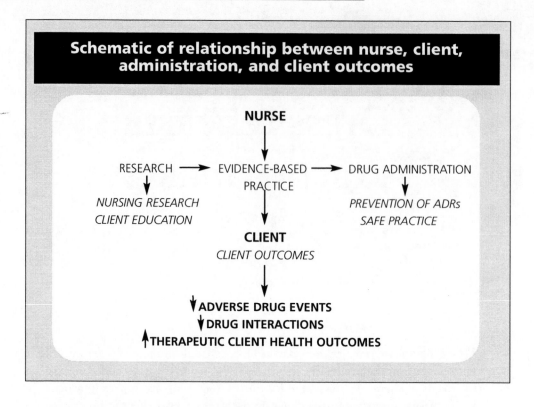

Break down barriers and deliver a strong performance

One barrier to effective practice is thinking you know more than you do. Think of this adage: "If you can't show it, you don't know it." The nurse who thinks he or she knows the details of a client's drug without doing the appropriate drug research is a classic example. Nothing takes the place of doing the actual legwork required, such as looking up the drugs for therapeutic action, side effects, clinical management, and cross-checking for drug interactions with other drugs on the client's medication list.

Another example of a barrier is only researching a particular piece of the drug information, such as researching clinical management without reviewing how to administer the drug, the expected side effects, and the drug interactions.

A third barrier is asking another nurse colleague to act as your drug surveyor. Interviewing your peers about drugs is not an acceptable drug reference. There are easily accessible, evidence-based nursing drug references, electronic databases, and pharmaceutical inserts to explore in an expert manner.

Find your own voice

Every nurse has his or her own practice style, from organizing a shift report and prioritizing an assignment to developing a timeline and demonstrating critical thinking by ordering what to do first. With drug administration, you will organize how many clients need to receive medications, which type, the time needed for preparation, equipment needed, and time needed for drug research. Despite barcoding and other electronic computer-assisted devices, you are still accountable for administering the right drugs to the right client, in the right dose, through the right route, and at the right time.

 Click: For more information on applications in evidence-based practice in nursing, click on these links:

www.nursingsociety.org/research/main.html#ebp
www.nursezone.com/Stories/SpotlightOnNurses.asp?articleID=12742

> *"A discovery is said to be an accident meeting a prepared mind."*
>
> —Albert Szent-Gyorgyi

Chapter 21

Evidence-based practice vs. *Alice in Wonderland*

Actors can participate in their own stunts and become characters in their own fantasy worlds, improvising with intuition and creativity. But nurses must be grounded in sound practice performances based on scientific evidence and cutting-edge research. No one wants a nurse who is like Alice in Wonderland. Clients expect nurses to be knowledgeable, safe, and have expert clinical practice and communication skills.

According to researchers, evidence-based medicine (EBM) is described as "the conscientious, explicit, and judicious use of current best evidence in making decisions about the care of individual patients" (Sackett et al.1996). "It is a method of solving clinical problems that stresses the examination of clinical research rather than relying on intuition and clinical experience alone" (Gordon and Rennie 2002).

Research your role

The nursing profession highly regards scholarship and the pursuit of innovations that enhance partnerships between nurses and clients, groups, communities, and other healthcare professionals. According to Sigma Theta Tau International, the honor society of nursing, "evidence-based nursing is an integration of the best evidence available, nursing expertise, and the values and preferences of individuals, families and communities who are served."

Evidence-based nursing requires that application of interventions be based on best practices supported by research, clinical expertise, and that are aligned with client preferences. Along with these essential components, all nurses can participate in the monitoring and evaluation of practice outcomes for clients, groups, and communities.

Action! Put your skills to the test

Nurses demonstrate the application of evidence-based practice every day. Decision-making and critical thought are essential. Based on what you have learned thus far about evidence-based practice in nursing, check *Yes* or *No* to the following activities nurses perform for drug administration. Which ones exemplify evidence-based practice?

		Yes	No
1.	Taking a client's pulse prior to administration of Digoxin 0.25 mg PO q AM.	___	___
2.	Giving a client water with medication.	___	___
3.	Calling the pharmacist and asking about a drug.	___	___
4.	Looking up coumadin 5 mg PO q PM for drug interactions in a nursing drug reference book.	___	___
5.	Becoming a nurse researcher.	___	___
6.	Following the nursing policy for drug administration that is on the intranet for that institution.	___	___

Answers:

1. Taking the client's pulse prior to administration of a cardiac glycoside such as Digoxin is performing an assessment based on evidence practice. Drug resources state to check the client's apical pulse prior to administration.

2. Giving the client water with medication is not based on evidence practice in this statement. If the nurse researched the drug with a drug reference prior to administration regarding whether to

administer the drug with water or food, then this would be an example of evidence-based practice.

3. Calling the pharmacist may be warranted and a good decision, but the information is just the pharmacist's opinion until the nurse verifies the reference from which the answer came.

4. Researching medications in drug references is practicing evidence-based interventions.

5. Becoming a nurse researcher is a great endeavor, but in and of itself, it is not evidence-based practice.

6. Nursing policies are based on research and evidence-based practice. References should be available that validate that the interventions stated in policies are research based.

Click: For further information on evidence-based practice, check out these resources:

www.ahrq.gov/clinic/jhppl/havighurst1.htm
www.acestar.uthscsa.edu/Resources_www.htm
http://evidence.ahc.umn.edu/ebn.htm
www.nsna.org/pubs/imprint/jan06/Jan06_FeatureBrown_Andereson.pdf

> *"Research is formalized curiosity. It is poking and prying with a purpose."*
>
> —Zora Neale Hurston

Chapter 22

Keep drug inserts off the cutting-room floor

Moving along with our movie, if an actor misplaces his script, he is lost! All his notes, suggestions, and prompts are necessary so he won't miss a cue. Nurses have their scripts, too, including the drug inserts that accompany medications. Sometimes information placed inside the box by drug manufacturers may not be easily accessible in other references. Drug inserts contain vital information from the drug manufacturer, including special handling and administration directions.

According to the U.S. Food and Drug Administration (FDA), each year, approximately 300,000 preventable adverse events occur in hospitals in this country, many as a result of confusing medical information. In January 2006, the FDA unveiled a major revision in the format of prescription drug information, commonly referred to as the package insert. This revision is the first in more than 25 years. The new format includes the reorganization of critical information.

Check out the new release

Changes in the format are targeted to make information about the drugs more accessible and include

- a new section called *Highlights* to provide immediate access to the most important prescribing information including boxed warnings, indications and usage, dosage, and administration

- a *Table of Contents* for easy reference to outline detailed safety and efficacy information

- the *date of initial product approval* so health professionals are made aware of how long the product has been on the market

- a new *patient counseling* section to emphasize communication between healthcare professionals and patients

- additional information including *use in specific populations, dosage forms and strengths, dosage and administration, contraindications, drug interactions,* and *adverse reactions*

- a *toll-free phone number for patients or doctors* to report suspected side effects to the FDA

These format and labeling changes to drug insert information have emerged based on the need to reduce the number of adverse drug events.

Here is the new look of drug information inserts:

Highlights of Prescribing Information

These highlights do not include all the information needed to use Imdicon safely and effectively. See full prescribing information for Imdicon.

IMDICON® (cholinasol) CAPSULES
Initial U.S. Approval: 2000

WARNING: LIFE-THREATENING HEMATOLOGICAL ADVERSE REACTIONS

See full prescribing information for complete boxed warning.
Monitor for hematological adverse reactions every 2 weeks for first 3 months of treatment (5.2). Discontinue Imdicon immediately If any of the following occur:

- **Neutropenia/agranulocytosis (5.1)**
- **Thrombotic thrombocytopenic purpura (5.1)**
- **Aplastic anemia (5.1)**

RECENT MAJOR CHANGES

Indications and Usage, Coronary Stenting (1.2)   2/200X
Dosage and Administration, Coronary Stenting (2.2)   2/200X

INDICATIONS AND USAGE

Imdicon is an adenosine diphosphate (ADP) antagonist platelet aggregation inhibitor indicated for:

- Reducing the risk of thrombotic stroke in patients who have experienced stroke precursors or who have had a completed thrombotic stroke (1.1)
- Reducing the incidence of subacute coronary stent thrombosis, when used with aspirin (1.2)

Important limitations:

- For stroke, Imdicon should be reversed for patients who are intolerant of or allergic to aspirin or who have failed aspirin therapy (1.1)

DOSAGE AND ADMINISTRATION

- Stroke: 50 mg once daily with food (2.1)
- Coronary Stenting: 50 mg once daily with food, with antiplatelet doses of aspirin, for up to 30 days following stent implantation (2.2) Discontinue in renally impaired patients if hemorrhagic or hematopoietic problems are encountered (2.3, 8.6, 12.3)

Highlights of Prescribing Information (cont.)

DOSAGE FORMS AND STRENGTH

Capsules: 50 mg (3)

CONTRAINDICATIONS

- Hematopoietic disorders or a history of TTP or aplastic anemia (4)
- Hemostatic disorder or active bleeding (4)
- Severe hepatic impairment (4,8,7)

WARNINGS AND PRECAUTIONS

- Neutropenia (2.4% of incidence; may occur suddenly; typically resolves within 1-2 weeks of discontinuation), thrombotic thrombocytopenic purpura (TTP), aplastic anemia, agranulocytosis, pancytopenia, leukemia, and thrombocytopenia can occur (5.1)
- Monitor for hematological adverse reactions every 2 weeks through the third month of treatment (5.2)

ADVERSE REACTIONS

Most common adverse reactions (incidence >2%) are diarrhea, nausea, dyspepsia, rash, gastrointestinal pain, neutropenia, and purpura (6.1)

To report SUSPECTED ADVERSE REACTIONS, contact (manufacturer) at (phone # and Web address) or FDA at 1-800-FDA-1088 or www.fda.gov/medwatch

DRUG INTERACTIONS

- Anticoagulants: Discontinue prior to switching to Imdicon (5.3, 7.1)
- Phenytoin: Elevated phenytoin levels have been reported. Monitor levels (7.2)

USE IN SPECIFIC POPULATIONS

- Hepatic impairment: Dose may need adjustment. Contraindicated in severe hepatic disease (4, 8.7, 12.3)
- Renal impairment: Dose may need adjustment. (2.3, 8.6, 12.3)

See 17 for PATIENT COUNSELING INFORMATION and FDA-approved patient labeling

Revised 5/200X

Source: Food & Drug Administration (www.fda.gov).

Ask: A nursing instructor was checking a new type of insulin with the nursing student assigned to the client. The primary nurse popped out of the client's room and stated that the medication could be combined with another type of insulin. The nursing instructor recommended that the nursing student check the insert in the box for mixing information. The drug insert stated, *Do not mix glargine (Lantus) with other insulins.* Following the correct way to approach drug administration through evidence-based research, the nursing instructor and student found out that it was not appropriate to combine that particular kind of insulin. The primary nurse had been giving the medication incorrectly. The nursing instructor and student showed the drug insert to the primary nurse, who stated that she did not know that the drug should not be mixed. What should the primary nurse have done before administering any medication?

Click: For further information regarding the new FDA drug insert labeling modifications, check out these resources:
www.fda.gov/bbs/topics/news/2005/NEW01272.html
www.fda.gov/cder/regulatory/physLabel/Imdicon.pdf
www.fda.gov/cder/regulatory/physLabel/physLabel_consumer.pdf

> "Do not go where the path may lead; go instead
> where there is no path and leave a trail."
>
> —Ralph Waldo Emerson

Chapter 23

The closing credits

Now that you have completed your journey through *Stressed Out About Drug Interactions,* you are ready to venture out on your own. As a professional nurse, you will implement the practices and strategies that were laid out for you throughout this book. Visualize yourself administering your client's medication, demonstrating expert preparation with prior evaluation of the drug research and evidence-based practice.

Remember, you are the heroes and heroines in this movie about safe drug administration. Deliver your Oscar-winning performances and your clients will remember you for your outstanding practice. Role model for others, so that you can make your mark on the nursing profession. Rave reviews from your clients, their families, and other professionals will soon follow. Stay your course, remain enthusiastic, have fun, make a commitment to life-long learning, and make your story one of safe nursing practice. Best of luck to you!

Part Four

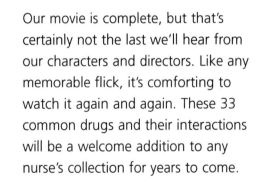

Our movie is complete, but that's certainly not the last we'll hear from our characters and directors. Like any memorable flick, it's comforting to watch it again and again. These 33 common drugs and their interactions will be a welcome addition to any nurse's collection for years to come.

Drugs list

 amoxicillin

Amoxil, Dispermox, Polymox, Sumox, Tri-mox, Wymox

Classification: Aminopenicillin
Therapeutic uses: Antibiotic, Antiulcer

Incompatible drugs/interaction effect
Allopurinol (↑ frequency of rash); aminoglycosides [{amikacin, gentamicin} ↓ efficacy]; cholestyramine, colestipol (↓ efficacy); methotrexate (↑ methotrexate toxicity); macrolides (erythromycin) ↓ efficacy; **oral contraceptives [{ethinyl estradiol, norelgestromin, norethindrone, norgestrel}↓ contraceptive efficacy]; probenecid (↓ renal excretion and ↑ blood levels of amoxicillin); **tetracyclines [{demeclocycline, doxycycline, minocycline}↓ efficacy]; warfarin (↑ effectiveness and ↑ risk of bleeding).

Food/beverages
May be taken with a small amount of food or beverage. Alcohol ↑ risk of stomach irritation.

Incompatible herbs/interaction effect
Bormelain (↑ efficacy and levels of amoxicillin).

Lab test interactions
May ↑ serum alkaline phosphatase, LDH, AST, and ALT.

Clinical management

PO; administer immediately after mixing. Shake oral suspension and use immediately. May be administered with or without food. Use 2 tsp. of water to dissolve Dispermox tablets, then ingest. Do not chew or swallow tablets. Chewable tablets should be chewed before drinking liquids. Advise client to report signs of anaphlyaxis (shortness of breath; swelling of face, life, tongue; or closing of throat). Notify healthcare provider for hives, severe watery diarrhea, unusual bleeding or bruising.

* Severity of reaction indicated by: * moderate, ** severe

ampicillin

Amcill, Ampicin, Omnipen, Penbritin, Principen, Polycillin, Totacillin

Classification: Aminopenicillin
Therapeutic uses: Antibiotic

Incompatible drugs/interaction effect

Allopurinol (↑ incidence ampicillin rash); aminoglycosides [{amikacin, gentamicin} ↓ efficacy]; atenolol (↓ efficacy); **contraceptives [{ethinyl estradiol, norelgestromin, norethindrone, norgestrel}↓ contraceptive efficacy]; chloramphenicol (↓ efficacy); erythromycin (↓ efficacy); gentamycin (↓ efficacy); *lansoprazole (↓ efficacy); *omeprazole (↓ ampicillin bioavailability); probenecid (↑ blood levels of ampicillin); tetracycline (↓ efficacy); warfarin (↑ risk of bleeding).

Food/beverages

With food, decreased ampicillin concentrations. Food may reduce efficacy by 25%–50%.

Incompatible herbs/interaction effect

Bormelain (↑ efficacy and levels of ampicillin).

Y-site incompatibility

Amphotericin B, epinephrine, fluconazole, hydralazine, midazolam, ondansetron, verapamil.

Syringe incompatibility

Erythromycin, gentamycin, kanamycin, metoclopramide.

114

Incompatible IV fluids

D5W, D5NS, D10W, fat emulsion 10%, LR, TPN, variable stability in NS.

Lab test interactions

Possible false positive reaction with urinary glucose tests with cupric sulfate (Benedict's solution, Clinitest).

Clinical management

PO; administer on empty stomach or at least one-half hour before meals or two hours after meals. Atenolol (monitor blood pressure and adjust dose); oral contraceptives (additional contraceptives should be used). Advise client to report signs of anaphlyaxis (shortness of breath; swelling of face, life, tongue; or closing of throat). Notify healthcare provider for hives, severe watery diarrhea, unusual bleeding or bruising.

* Severity of reaction indicated by: * moderate, ** severe

atenolol

Tenormin

Classification: Beta-adrenergic antagonist, sympatholytic blocking agent
Therapeutic uses: Antihypertensive

Incompatible drugs/interaction effect

Alcohol (↑ efficacy); **amiodarone (↑ hypotension, bradycardia and cardiac arrest), **albuterol (↓ effectiveness of beta adrenergic blockers/beta-2 agonist); ** anti-diabetic drugs [{acrabose, acetohexamide, chlorpropamide, glimepiride, glipizide, glyburide, metformin, repaglinide, tolazamide, tolbutamide}↑ hypoglycemia, hyperglycemia, hypertension]; alpha-1 blockers [{phenoxybenzamine, phento-lamine, prazosin, terazosin} ↑ hypotension first dose); **ampicillin (↓ efficacy for lowering blood pressure and treating angina); **calcium channel blockers [{amlodipine, disopyramide, diltiazem, felodipine, nicardipine, nifedipine} ↑ brady-cardia and/or hypotension, ↓ cardiac output]; calcium (↓ efficacy); chlorpromazine (↑ hypotension and/or phenothiazine toxicity); **digoxin (↑ bradycardia, AV block and possible digoxin toxicity); fentanyl (severe hypotension); general anes-thesia: [{IV phenytoin and verapamil} ↑ myocardial depression]; **lidocaine (↑ lidocaine level and risk for toxicity); metaproterenol (↓ efficacy of beta-adrenergic blocker/beta-2 agonist); methyldopa (↑ hypertension, tachycardia, arrhythmias); *NSAIDs [{etodolac, diclofenac, diflunisal, ketorolac, ibuprofen, indomethacin, naproxen, piroxicam} ↓ efficacy for lowering blood pressure]; *prazosin (↑ risk of orthostatic hypotension); *quinidine (↑ efficacy beta-blocker); *salicylates [{aspirin, bismuth subsalicylate, sodium salicylate} ↓ efficacy of beta-blockers]; salmeterol (↓ effectiveness of beta adrenergic blockers/beta-2 agonist); **verapamil (↑ efficacy of atenolol and ↑ efficacy of verapamil).

Food/beverages
May interact with orange juice.

Incompatible herbs/interaction effect
Dong Quai (↑ hypotensive response to first dose of alpha blocker); guar gum (↑ hypoglycemia, hyperglycemia, hypertension); Ma huang (↓ hypotensive effect of beta-adrenergic blocker); St. John's wort (↓ efficacy of beta-adrenergic blockers); Yohimbine (↓ efficacy of beta-adrenergic blockers).

Y-site incompatibility
Amphotericin B.

Lab test interactions
May cause ↑ BUN, potassium, triglycerides, serum lipoprotein, and uric acid levels.

Clinical management
Monitor client's blood pressure and assess for angina. Separate doses to ↓ incidence of interaction. ✓ for normal therapeutic level of lidocaine (2 to 5 mcg/mL). Assess for lidocaine toxicity (dizziness, somnolence, confusion, parethesias, seizures). Salicylates; monitor client for signs and symptoms of heart failure and hypertension. Verapamil: Monitor for ↑ heart failure, left ventricular dysfunction, and AV conduction defects. ↑ risk of interaction with IV administration. Advise client to check BP periodically. Advise client to check with healthcare provider before taking any other medication. Client should report dizziness, fainting, confusion, chest pains, irregular heart beat, or swelling in hands, legs, or feet immediately.

PO
Take on empty stomach. Do not miss doses, but if missed take immediately up to 8 hours before next dose. **Do not stop abruptly** (may precipitate life-threatening arrhythmias, hypertension, myocardial ischemia).

* Severity of reaction indicated by: * moderate, ** severe

cephalexin

Bio-Cef, Keflex, Keftab, Panixine DisperDose

Classification: First Generation Cepholasporin
Therapeutic uses: Anti-infective, antibiotic

Incompatible drugs/interaction effect

Aminoglycosides (↑ nephrotoxicity); *Cholestyramine (↓ efficacy); metformin (↑ plasma levels); probenecid (↓ renal excretion of cephalexin).

Food/beverages

↓ delayed serum peak but does not affect total absorption.

Lab test interactions

Prolonged prothrombin time may ↑ BUN, creatinine, alkaline phosphatase, bilirubin, LDH levels. May cause positive direct Coombs', false-positive urinary glucose test using cupric sulfate (Benedict's solution, Clinitest, Fehling's solution), false-positive serum or urine creatinine with Jaffé reaction, false-positive urinary proteins and steroids.

Clinical management

PO; refrigerate oral suspension. Shake well prior to use. Take with food or milk to prevent gastrointestinal upset. Use 2 tsp. of water to dissolve Dispermox tablets, then ingest. Do not chew or swallow tablets. Advise client to report rash, severe diarrhea, decreased urine output, or unusual bleeding or bruising to healthcare providers.

* Severity of reaction indicated by: * moderate, ** severe

cefazolin sodium

Acef, Kefzol, Zolicef

Classification: First Generation Cepholasporin
Therapeutic uses: Anti-infective, antibiotic

Incompatible drugs/interaction effect

Probenecid (↓ renal excretion of cefazolin ↑ blood levels); *Warfarin (↑ risk of bleeding); Use together with loop diuretics or aminoglycosides ↑ nephrotoxicity.

Y-site incompatibility

Ascorbic acid (precipitate); aminoglycosides; amiodarone (precipitate); amphotericin B cholesteryl sulfate, cimetidine (precipitate); idarubicin, pentamidine, TPN. Vancomycin (concentration dependent); vinorelbine.

Lab test considerations

May ↑ ALT, AST, alkaline phosphatase, BUN, creatinine levels. May cause positive direct Coombs', false-positive urinary glucose test using cupric sulfate (Benedict's solution, Clinitest, Fehling's solution), false-positive serum or urine creatinine with Jaffé reaction.

Clinical management

For IV infusion, administer over 30–60 minutes. Notify healthcare provider for severe diarrhea, decreased urine output, or unusual bleeding or bruising.

* Severity of reaction indicated by: * moderate, ** severe

ciprofloxacin

Cipro, Cirpro XR, Proquin XR

Classification: Fluoroquinolone
Therapeutic uses: Antibiotic, anti-infective

gatifloxacin (Tequin)
gemifloxacin (Factive)
levofloxacin (Levaquin)
lomefloxacin (Maxaquin)
moxifloxacin (Avelox)
norfloxacin (Noroxin)
ofloxacin (Floxin)
sparfloxacin (Zagam)

Incompatible drugs/interaction effect

↑ risk of serious cardiovascular events with concurrent use of amiodarone, disopyramide, erythromycin, gatifloxacin, gemifloxacin, moxifloxacin, pentamidine, phenothiazines, pimozide, procainamide, quinidine, sotalol, sparfloxacin, tricyclic antidepressants. ↑ theophylline levels may result in toxicity. Probenecid

(↑ serum ciprofloxacin level). *NSAIDs with high doses of quinolones has precipitated seizures in pre-clinical studies.

↓ absorption with antacids, bismuth subsalicylate, iron salts {(ferrous fumarate, ferrous gluconate, ferrous sulfate) ↓ efficacy}, sucralfate (↓ gastrointestinal absorption) and zinc salts. ↓ fluoroquinolone serum levels by antineoplastics. ↓ elmination with cimetidine. ↑ seizures with foscarnet. ↑ risk of spontaneous tendon rupture with corticosteroids, ↑ risk of hypoglycemia with antidiabetics.

Food/beverages
↓ absorption with concurrent tube feeding. Ciprofloxacin should not be taken with milk or yogurt alone but may be taken with other dietary calcium foods. ↓ absorption of norfloxacin with food/diary products.

Incompatible herbs/interaction effect
Fennel (↓ absorption of ciprofloxacin); St. John's Wort (↑ photosensitivity).

Y-site incompatibility
Ciprofloxacin; **do not mix with other solutions.** Flush before and after administration (aminophylline, ampicillin/sulbactam, azithromycin, dexamethasone, furosemide, heparin, hydrocortisone, methylprednisolone, phenytoin, potassium phosphates, propofol, sodium phosphates, warfarin). Gatifloxacin; **do not mix with other solutions.** Flush before and after administration (amphotericin B, cefoperazone, cefoxitin, diazepam, furosemide, heparin, phenytoin, piperacillin, piperacillin/tazobactam, potassium phosphates, vancomycin). Levofloxacin; **do not mix with other solutions.** Flush before and after administration (acyclovir, alprostadil, azithromycin, furosemide, heparin, indomethacin, nitroglycerin, nitroprusside, propofol). Moxifloxacin; **do not mix with other solutions.** Flush before and after administration. Ofloxacin; **do not mix with other solutions.** Flush before and after administration (amphotericin B, cholesteryl sulfate, cefepime, doxorubicin).

Clinical management
PO; administer at least 2 hours from calcium, iron, or zinc. PO; administer at least 6 hours after ciprofloxacin. Administer 1 hour before or 2 hours after food/diary products. Extended release form may be taken with meals with diary products. Advise client to stay out of sun while on this medication to avoid photosensitivity reaction. Client should report confusion, fainting, irregular heart beat, joint or muscle pain, numbness, tingling or loss of muscle strength.

* Severity of reaction indicated by: * moderate, ** severe

clindamycin

Cleocin, Cleocin T, Clinda-Derm, Clindagel, Clindesse, ClindaMax, Clindets, C/T/S, Evoclin

Classification: Lincosamide

Therapeutic uses: Antibiotic, anti-infective

Incompatible drugs/interaction effect

*Cyclosporin (↓ cyclosporin bioavailability); **erythromycin (antagonistic antimicrobial effects and/or ↑ risk of cardiotoxicity); nondepolarizing muscle relaxants (*atacurium, *mivacurium, *pancuronium, *rocuronium, *vecuronium, ↑ efficacy).

Food/beverages

Kaolin/Pectin ↓ gastrointestinal absorption; food may delay peak concentrations.

Incompatible herbs/interaction effect

St. John's Wort may ↓ clindamycin levels.

Y-site incompatibility

Allopurinol, azithromycin, ceftriaxone, ciprofloxacin, filgrastim, flucoazole, idarubicin, Phenobarbital, phenytoin.

Syringe incompatibility

Tobramycin.

Lab test interactions

May cause transient decreases in leukocytes, eosinophils and platelets. May cause elevations in alkaline phosphatase, bilirubin, CPK, AST, and ALT.

Clinical management

PO; give with full glass of water. May be given with food. Client should report loose stools or diarrhea immediately to healthcare provider. Too rapid IV infusions have precipitated hypotension and cardiopulmonary arrest.

* Severity of reaction indicated by: * moderate, ** severe

coumadin

Coumadin, Warfilone, Warfarin

Classification: Courmarins
Therapeutic uses: Anticoagulant

Incompatible drugs/interaction effect

**Abciximab (↑ risk of bleeding); *acarbose (↑ risk of bleeding); ** aceno-coumarol (↑ risk of bleeding); *acetaminophen (↑ risk of bleeding); *alclofenac (↑ risk of bleeding); **alteplase (↑ risk of bleeding); *amiodarone (↑ risk of bleeding); *amitriptyline (↑ risk of bleeding); *amoxapine (↑ risk of bleeding); *amoxicillin (↑ risk of bleeding); ** aspirin (↑ risk of bleeding); *atenolol (↑ prothrombin time or international normalized ratio (INR); *azathioprine (↓ anticoagulant efficacy); *azithromycin (↑ risk of bleeding); *bismuth subsalicylate (↑ risk of bleeding); *capecitabine (↑ risk of bleeding); *carbamazebine (↓ anticoagulant efficacy); *cefamandole (↑ risk of bleeding); *cefazolin (↑ risk of bleeding); *cefoperazone (↑ risk of bleeding); *cefotetan (↑ risk of bleeding); **celecoxib (↑ risk of bleeding); *chloral hydrate (↑ risk of bleeding); *choramphenicol (↑ risk of bleeding); *chlordiazepoxide (↑ risk of bleeding); *chlorpromazine (↓ efficacy of warfarin); *cholestyramine (↓ efficacy of warfarin); **cilostazol (↑ risk of bleeding); *cimetidine (↑ risk of bleeding); *ciprofloxacin (↑ risk of bleeding); *cisapride (↑ risk of bleeding); *clarithromycin (↑ risk of bleeding); *clofibrate (↑ risk of bleeding); *clomipramine (↑ risk of bleeding); *clopidogrel (↑ risk of bleeding); *cloxacillin (↑ risk of bleeding); *cyclosporine (↓ anticoagulant and cyclosporine efficacy); **dalteparin (↑ risk of bleeding); **danazol (↑ risk of bleeding); *despiramine (↑ risk of bleeding); *diazoxide (↑ anticoagulant and ↑ risk of bleeding): *dicloxacillin (↓ risk anticoagulant efficacy): * dicumarol (↑ risk of bleeding); * diflusinal (↑ risk of bleeding); *diospyramide (↑ risk of bleeding); *disulfiram (↑ risk of bleeding); *doxepin (↑ risk of bleeding); *doxycycline (↑ risk of bleeding); *erythromycin (↑ risk of bleeding); *esomeprazole (↑ INR and ↑ anticoagulant efficacy); *ethacrynic acid (↑ risk of bleeding); *oral contraceptives (↑ or ↓ anticoagulant efficacy); fluconazole (↑ risk of bleeding); *fluorouracil(↑ risk of bleeding); *fluoxetine (↑ risk of bleeding); *fluvastatin (↑ risk of bleeding); *gatifloxacin, gemifloxacin (↑ risk of bleeding); *gemfibrozil (↑ risk of bleeding); *glipizide (↑ risk of hypoglycemia); *glucagon (↑ risk of bleeding); *glyburide (↑ risk of bleeding); **heparin (↑ risk of bleeding); *isoniazid (↑ risk of bleeding);* itraconazole, *ketocaconazole (↑ risk of bleeding); *lactulose (↑ INR and ↑ anticoagulant efficacy); *lansoprazole (↑ INR and anticoagulant efficacy); *levofloxacin (↑ risk of bleeding); *levothyroxine (↑ risk of bleeding); *liothyronine (↑ risk of bleeding); * lovastatin (↑ risk of bleeding); *menthol (↓ anticoagulant efficacy); *methylphenidate (↑ serum warfarin levels and risk of bleeding); *methylprednisolone (↑ risk of bleeding and ↓ anticoagulant effects); *metronidazole (↑ risk of bleeding); *miconazole (↑ risk of bleeding); *minocycline (↑ risk of bleeding); *nafcillin (↓ anticoagulant efficacy); *norfloxacin (↑ risk of bleeding); *nortriptyline (↑ risk of bleeding); *NSAIDs [{acemetacin, benoxaprofen, bromfenac, carprofen, diclofenac, dipyrone, enoxacin, etodolac, felbamate, fenbufen, fenofibrate, fenoprofen, ibuprofen, indomethacin, indoprofen, isoxicam, ketoprofen, ketorolac, meclofenamate, meloxicam, moxalactam, nabumetone, oxaprozin, oxyphenbutazone, phenylbutazone, pirazolac, piroxicam, propyphenazone, ** naproxen; tenoxicam, tolmetin}↑ risk of bleeding]; *ofloxacin (↑ risk of bleeding); *omeprazole (↑ INR and ↑ anticoagulant efficacy); *paroxetine (↑ risk of bleeding); **phenidione (↑ risk of bleeding); *phenobarbital (↓ anticoagulant efficacy); *phenytoin (↑ risk of bleeding); *potassium iodide (↓ anticoagulant efficacy); *propafenone (↑ risk of bleeding); *proproxyphene (↑ risk of bleeding); *propranolol (↑ risk of bleeding); *propylthiouracil (↓ anticoagulant efficacy); *Protease Inhibitors [{amprenavir (↑ anticoagulant efficacy), atazanavir (↑ risk of bleeding); darunavir (altered anticoagulant concentration); fosamprenavir (↑ warfarin serum concentrations), nevirapine (↓ anticoagulant efficacy), reviparin (↑ risk of bleeding), ritonavir (↓ serum warfarin concentrations), saquinavir (↑ risk of bleeding;] *quinidine (↑ risk of bleeding); *quinine (↑ risk of bleeding); raloxifene (↓ anticoagulant efficacy); *ranitidine (↑ risk of bleeding); *rifabutin (↓ warfarin efficacy); *rifapin (↓ anticoagulant efficacy); *sertraline (↑ risk of bleeding); *simvastatin (↑ risk of bleeding); *spironolactone (↓ anticoagulant efficacy); *sulcrafate (↓ warfarin efficacy); *sulfamethoxazole (↑ risk of bleeding); **sulfisoxazole ↑ risk of bleeding); *sulindac (↑ risk of bleeding); **tamoxifen (↑ risk of bleeding); *tetracycline (↑ risk of bleeding); *ticlopidine (↑ risk of bleeding); *tramadol (↑ PT and risk of bleeding); *vancomycin (↑ risk of bleeding); *vitamin A (↑ risk of bleeding); vitamin E (↑ risk of bleeding); zafirlukast (↑ risk of bleeding).

Food/beverages

Alcohol (↓ or ↑ INR); avocado (↓ anticoagulant efficacy); ↓ efficacy foods high in vitamin K; **↑ cranberry juice (↑ risk of bleeding and efficacy); high-protein foods (↓ efficacy); papaya (↑ risk of bleeding); pumpkin seed. (↑ risk of bleeding); soybean (↓ warfarin efficacy). Foods high in vitamin K interfere with anticoagulant efficacy {alfalfa, asparagus, broccoli, brussels sprouts, cabbage, cauliflower, green teas, kale, lettuce, spinach, turnip greens, watercress, beef liver, pork liver, green tea, and green leafy vegetables.

Incompatible herbs/interaction effect

*Anise (↑ risk of bleeding); *bilberry (↑ risk of bleeding); *capsaicin (↑ risk of bleeding); *cat's claw (↑ risk of bleeding); *celery (↑ risk of bleeding); *chamomile (↑ risk of bleeding); *chondroitin (↑ INR and ↑ anticoagulant efficacy); *coenzyme Q10 (↑ anticoagulant efficacy); *devil's claw (↑ risk of bleeding); *Dong Quai (↑ risk of bleeding); **garlic (↑ risk of bleeding); *ginger (↑ risk of bleeding); **ginseng (↑ INR and anticoagulant efficacy); *glucosamine (↑ INR and anticoagulant efficacy); *green tea (↑ anticoagulant efficacy); *kava (↑ risk of bleeding); *licorice (↑ risk of bleeding); *melatonin (↑ risk of bleeding); *saw palmetto (↑ risk of bleeding); St. John's wort (↑ serum warfarin and ↓ anticoagulant efficacy).

Y-site incompatibility

Aminophylline, bretylium, ceftazidime, cimetidime, ciprofloxacin, dobutamine, esmolol, gentamicin, labetalol, metronidazole, promazine, vancomycin.

Syringe incompatibility

Heparin.

Incompatible IV fluids

Variable compatibility lactated ringers (LR), normal saline (NS).

Clinical management

Monitor INR and PT for therapeutic values and to prevent hemorrhage. Advise client not to change brands because bioavailabilites are not equivalent. Monitor for signs of hemorrhage or thrombosis. Tell the client to immediately report any signs and symptoms of bleeding (gums, nosebleed, tarry stools, hematuria, heavy menstrual flow) to healthcare provider. Monitor CBC, PT-INR, AST, ALT throughout therapy. Advise client to check with healthcare provider before taking any other medications. Provide client education regarding foods high in vitamin K, which decrease efficacy of anticoagulants.

* Severity of reaction indicated by: * moderate, ** severe

digoxin
Digitek, Lanoxin, Lanoxicaps

Classification: Cardiac glycoside
Therapeutic uses: Antiarrhythmic, inotropic

Incompatible drugs/interaction effect
**Amiodarone (digoxin toxicity); amphotericin B (hypokalemia and ↑ digoxin toxicity); antacids [{aluminum carbonate, aluminum hyrdroxide, magnesium carbonate, magnesium hydroxide, magnesium oxide} ↓ digoxin levels and efficacy]; antidiabetic drugs [{*acarbose, *metoclopramide, metformin (↑ metformin level)} (↓ efficacy]; *beta-adrenergic blockers [{acebutolol, atenolol, carteolol, carvedilol, esmolol, labetalol, metoprolol, propranolol, sotalol} AV block and ↑ digoxin toxicity]; **benzadiazepines [{alprazolam, diazepam, ↑ efficacy and digoxin toxicity}]; **calcium(arrhythmia and cardiovascular collapse); calcium channel blockers [{diltiazem, ↑ digoxin serum levels and toxicity]; colestipol (↓ digoxin efficacy); cyclosporine (↑ digoxin toxicity); *disopyramide (↑ digoxin serum levels and toxicity diuretics); **doxycycline (↑ digoxin serum levels and toxicity); *diuretics [{acetazolamide, bumetanide, chlorothiazide, furosemide, **hydrochlorothiazide, hypokalemia and ↑ digoxin toxicity}; amiloride, [(↓ digoxin efficacy)]; *fluoxetine (↑ risk of digoxin toxicity); gatifloxacin (↑ risk of digoxin toxicity); **itraconazole (↑ risk of digoxin toxicity); *lansoprazole (↑ risk of digoxin toxicity); (↑ **Macrolides [{azithromycin, clarithromycin, erythromycin}↑ digoxin toxicity]; NSAIDS [{*diclofenac, *etodolac, ** indomethacin} ↑ digoxin toxicity]; omeprazole (↑ risk of digoxin toxicity); *statins [{atorvastatin, simvastatin}↑ efficacy and digoxin plasma levels}]; pipercillin (↑ risk of digoxin toxicity); **quinidine (digoxin toxicity); **quinine (digoxin toxicity); rifampin (↓ digoxin levels); ritonavir (↑ digoxin toxicity); **spironolactone (↑ risk of digoxin toxicity); *sulcrafate (↓ digoxin efficacy); **tetracycline (↑ digoxin levels and toxicity); ticarcillin (↑ risk of digoxin toxicity); *tramadol (↑ risk of digoxin toxicity); *trazodone (↑ risk of digoxin toxicity); *trimethroprim (↑ risk of digoxin toxicity); thyroid hormones (may ↓ therapeutic effects); **verapamil (digoxin toxicity).

Food/beverages
Foods high in fiber may decrease absorption.

Incompatible herbs/interaction effect
*Aloe (hypokalemia and ↑ digoxin toxicity); *carob (↑ digoxin toxicity); *cascara sagrada (hypokalemia and ↑ digoxin toxicity); ginseng (↑ digoxin toxicity);

*licorice (↑ digoxin toxicity); *senna (↑ digoxin toxicity); **St John's wort
(↓ digoxin efficacy).

Y-site incompatibility

Amiodarone, amphotericin B cholesteryl sulfate, fluconazole, foscarnet, propofol.

Syringe incompatibility

Manufacturer recommends that digoxin not be mixed with other drugs.

Clinical management

PO; administer medication 1 hour before or 2 hours after meals with high fiber.
Check BP regularly and take pulse prior to administration. Contact healthcare
provider if pulse is less than 60 or greater than 100. Monitor serum digoxin level
and potassium.

* Severity of reaction indicated by: * moderate, ** severe

diazepam

Diastat, Diazemuls, Dizac, D-Val, Valium

Classification: Benzodiazepine

Therapeutic uses: Antianxiety, anticonvulsant, sedative/hypnotic, skeletal muscle relaxant

Incompatible drugs/interaction effect

*Alcohol (↑ CNS effects); **alfentanil (↑ respiratory depression); amitriptyline
(↑ psychomotor deficits); *antifungals [{fluconazole, itraconazole, ketoconazole,
miconazole} ↑ CNS and benzodiazepine toxicity]; **carisoprodol (↑ respiratory
depression); **chloral hydrate (↑ respiratory depression); **chlorzoxazone (↑ respiratory depression); **codeine (↑ respiratory depression); *dalfopristin (↑ risk of
diazepam toxicity); *dantrolene (↑ respiratory depression); *digoxin (↑ digoxin
toxicity); disulfiram (↑ CNS depression); *macrolides [{clarithromycin, erythromycin, roxithromycin} ↑ sedative effects and benzodiazepine toxicity (CNS depres-
son, ataxia, lethargy)], **fentanyl (↑ respiratory depression); *fluvoxamine
(diazepam accumulation); **hydrocodone (↑ respiratory depression); **hydromorphone (↑ respiratory depression); isoniazid (↑ risk of benzodiazepine toxicity);
**levorphanol (↑ CNS depression); **meperidine (↑ respiratory depression);
**meprobamate (↑ respiratory depression); metaxalone (↑ respiratory depres-
sion); **methocarbamol (↑ respiratory depression); *mirtazapine (↑ impairment

of motor skills); **morphine (↑ respiratory depression); **oxycodone (↑ respiratory depression); **oxymorphone (↑ respiratory depression); *pentobarbital (↑ respiratory depression); **phenobarbital (↑ respiratory depression); *phenytoin (alteration of serum phenytoin levels); **proxyphene (↑ respiratory depression); *quinupristine (↑ risk of diazepam toxicity); *rifampin (↓ diazepam effacy); *protease inhibitors [{amprenavir, atazanavir, indinavir, lopinavir-ritonavir, nelfinavir, ritonavir, saquinavir} ↑ sedative effects leading to respiratory depression and ↑ risk of diazepam toxicity], **sufentanil (↑ respiratory depression); theophylline (↑ respiratory depression).

Food/beverages
Alcohol (↑ CNS depression and sedation); caffeine (↓ sedative and anxiolytic effects of diazepam); grapefruit juice (↑ plasma concentrations of diazepam); high-fat foods (↑ diazepam concentrations).

Incompatible herbs/interaction effect
↑ CNS depression with kava, valerian, or chamomile.

Y-site incompatibility
Amphotericin B cholesteryl sulfate, atacruium, cefepime, diltiazem, fluconazole, foscarnet, gatifloxacin, heparin, hydrocortisone, hydromorphone, linezolid, meropenem, pancuronium, potassium chloride, propofol, vecuronium, vitamin B complex with C.

Syringe incompatibility
Doxapram, glycopyrrolate, furosemide, heparin, hydromorphone, morphine, nalbuphine, sufentanil.

Incompatible IV fluids
Do not dilute or mix with any other drug. Do not use continuous infusion because of precipitation in IV fluids and absorption of diazepam into infusion bags and tubing. Check with pharmacy variable data regarding IV fluid compatibility.

Lab test interactions
May cause false-negative urinary glucose determinations when using Clinistix or Diastix.

Clinical management
Monitor for respiratory depression, bradycardia, hypotension and CNS depression. PO; may administer with food or water, and tablets can be crushed. Advise client

not to combine with alcohol or other CNS depressants. Consult with healthcare provider before combining with other medciations. IV: Rapid administration may result in apnea, hypotension, bradycardia, or cardiovascular collapse.

* Severity of reaction indicated by: * moderate, ** severe

diltiazem

Cardizem, Cardizem LA, CartiaXT, Dilacor XR, Diltia XT, Nu-Diltiaz, Syn-Diltiazem, Tiamate, Tiazac

Classification: Calcium Channel Blocker
Therapeutic uses: Antianginal, antiarrhythmic, antihypertensive

Incompatible drugs/interaction effect

Alcohol (↑ hypotension), amiodarone (bradycardia, atroventricular block/cardiac arrest); *aspirin (prolonged bleeding time); *benzodiazepines [{alprazolam, diazepam, midazolam, triazolam} ↑ bioavailability, sedation, efficacy}; *beta-blockers [{acebutolol, atenolol, betaxolol, carteolol, carvedilol, esmolol, metoprolol, nadolol, pinolol, propranolol, sotalol, timolol {bradycardia, conduction defects and CHF}]; *buspirone (↑ buspirone level), *carbamazepine (↑ carbamazepine level and risk of toxicity), cimetidine (↑ blood levels and efficacy), cyclosporine (↑ cyclosporine level and risk of toxicity), and cholestyramine (↓ diltiazem bioavailabilty); *cilostazol (↑ cilostazol side effects); cimetidine (↑ diltiazem concentrations and ↑ cardiovascular toxicity); *cisapride (contraindicated, risk of cardiotoxicity); *colestipol (↓ diltiazem bioavailability); *cyclosporine (↑ risk of cyclosporine toxicity); digoxin (↑ serum digoxin levels), disopyramide (bradycardia, conduction defects and CHF, *droperidol (↑ risk of cardiotoxicity); fentanyl (↑ hypotension), *erythromycin (↑ risk of cardiotoxicity); *fosphenytoin (↑ risk phenytoin toxicity); *HMG-CoA reductase inhibitors [{atorvastatin, lovastatin, simvastatin} ↑ HMG-CoA reductase level and risk of toxicity, ↑ risk of rhabdomyolysis}], *methylprednisolone (↑ methylprednisolone effects *risk of toxicity); *moricizine (↓ efficacy); *NSAIDs [{aceclofenac, acemetacin, alclofenac, apazone, benoxaprofen, bromfenac, celecoxib, clometacin, dalfopristin, diclofenac, diflunisal, droxicam, etodolac, etofenamate, felbinac, fenoprofen, flurbiprofen, ibuprofen, indomethacin, indoprofen, isoxicam, meclofenamate, meloxicam, nabumetone, naproxen, oxaprozin, oxyphenbutazone, phenylbutazone, pirazolac, piroxicam, propyphenazone, sulindac, tenoxicam, tolmetin} ↑ risk of gasterointestinal hemorrhage and ↓ efficacy of antihypertensive effects], **fentanyl (severe hypotension); **fentiazac (↑ risk of gastrointestinal hemorrhage/antagonism of hypotensive effect); phenytoin (bradycardia, conduction defects and CHF), *labetalol (↑ risk hypotension, bradycardia, AV conduction disturbances); *lithium (neurotoxicity, psychosis); *methylprednisolone (↑ methylprednisolone plasma level); *nifedipine (↑ nifedipine toxicity); *phenytoin (↑ risk of phenytoin toxicity); *protease inhibitors [{amprenavir, delavirdine, fosamprenavir, indinavir, nevirapine, ritonavir, saquinavir} ↑ serum diltiazem concentration and ↑ risk of cardiotoxicity]; *ranitidine (↑ blood levels and efficacy); quinidine (↑ quinidine effects and risk of toxicity); *quinupristin (↑ risk of diltiazem toxicity); *rifampin (↓ diltiazem efficacy); *tacrolimus (↑ tacrolimus level and risk of toxicity), *theophylline [{↑ theophylline level and risk of toxicity}].

Food/beverages
Alcohol (may ↑ risk of hypotension or vasodilation), food (↑ plasma concentrations), grapefruit juice (↑ serum diltiazem concentrations).

Incompatible herbs/interaction effect
*Ma huang (↓ hypotensive effect of diltiazem); St. John's wort (↓ bioavailability of diltiazem); yohimbine (↓ ditiazem efficacy).

Y-site incompatibility
Diazepam, furosemide, phenytoin, rifampin, thiopental. Manufacturer states do not mix IV product with other medications.

Lab test interactions
May cause ↑ transient increase in ALT, AST.

Clinical management
PO; may be administered with or without food. Sustained release forms should not be crushed, broken, or chewed to avoid overdose. Client should check with healthcare provider before taking any other medications. Monitor heart rate and blood pressure. Advise client to report dizziness, shortness of breath, peripheral edema, noisy respirations, weight gain, and chest pain. Client should hold medication and notify healthcare provider for low heart rate and blood pressure. Advise client for signs and symptoms of digoxin toxicity (confusion, weakness, dizziness, irregular heartbeat, loss of appetite, nausea, vomiting, abdominal distress, and changes in color vision, including seeing halos around lights.) Client should hold medication and notify healthcare provider for low heart rate and blood pressure.

* Severity of reaction indicated by: * moderate, ** severe

diphenhydramine

Banophen, Belix, Benadryl Dye Free Allergy, Benadryl Allergy, Benadryl, Benylin, Compoz, Compoz Nighttime Sleep Aid, Diphen AF, Diphen Cough, Diphenhist, Dormin, Genahist, 40 Winks, Hyrexin50, Insomnal, Maximum Strength Nytol, Maximum Sleepinal, Midol PM, Nighttime Sleep Aid, Nytol, Scot-Tussin Allergy DM, Siladryl, Silfphen DM, Sleepwell2-night, Sominex, Tusstat, Unisom Nighttime Sleep Aid.

Classification: H1-receptor antagonist

Therapeutic uses: Allergy, cold, cough remedy, antihistamine, antitussives

Incompatible drugs/interaction effect

Antihistamines, alcohol, *amitriptyline (↑ anticholinergic effects); clormipramine (↑ anticholinergic effects); metoprolol (↑ risk of metoprolol toxicity); opioid analgesics, sedative/hypnotics ↑ CNS depression, disopyramide, MAOIs, quinidine, tricyclic antidepressants ↑ anticholinergic effects.

Incompatible herbs/interaction effect

Kava, valerian, chamomile ↑ CNS depression.

Y-site incompatibility

Allopurinol, amphotericin B cholesteryl sulfate, cefepime, dilantin, foscarnet, furosemide.

Syringe incompatibility

Haloperidol, pentobarbital, thiopental.

Incompatible IV fluids

N/A

Lab test considerations

May decrease skin response to allergy testing.

Clinical management

Do not give by subcutaneous injection. PO; give with meals or milk to ↓ gastrointestinal irritation. Capsule may be emptied and taken with food or water. **Overdosage in infants and children can cause hallucinations, seizures, or death. Advise client that this medication causes drowsiness and to determine response before driving or operating machinery. Client should not combine with CNS depressants.

* Severity of reaction indicated by: * moderate, ** severe

epinephrine

Adrenalin, Ana-Guard, Asthma Haler Mist, AsthmaNefrin (racepinephrine, EpiPen, microNefrin, Primatene, Sus-Phrine, S-2

Classification: Adrenergic, alpha/beta agonist
Therapeutic uses: Antiasthmatics, bronchodilator, vasopressor, antidote

Incompatible drugs/interaction effect

Additive effect with other adrenergics. Hypertensive crisis with **MAOIs (isocarboxazid, phenelzine, tranylcpromine). ↑ response with *methyldopa (Aldomet), ↑ efficacy *tricyclic antidepressants [(amitriptyline, amoxapine, clomipramine, desipramine, doxepin, imipramine, nortriptyline, trimipramine); ↑ risk of hypertension and arrhythmias}]. **Beta-blockers [(carteolol, nadolol, penbutolol, pindolol, propranolol, timolol) {marked hyptensive effects followed by reflex bradycardia}].

Incompatible herbs/interaction effect

Yohimbine (↑ CNS stimulation).

Y-site incompatibility

Ampicillin, thiopental.

Additive incompatibility

Ampicillin, sodium bicarbonate.

Syringe incompatibility

Sodium bicarbonate.

Clinical management

High-alert comes in many different forms and concentrations.

* Severity of reaction indicated by: * moderate, ** severe

erythromycin

A/T/S, E-Base, E-Mycin, Erybid, Erythrocin, Eryc, Ery-Tab, PCE

Classification: Macrolide

Therapeutic uses: Antibiotic, anti-infective

Incompatible drugs/interaction effect

*Alfentanil (↓ alfentanil clearance); *alprazolam (↑ benzodiazepine toxicity);
**amiodarone (↑ risk cardiotoxicty); **amitriptyline (↑ risk of cardiotoxicity);
**amoxapine (↑ risk of cardiotoxicity); **atorvastatin (↑ atorvastatin and ↑ risk
of myopathy or rhabdomyolysis); **bretylium (↑ risk of cardiotoxicity); *buspirone
(↑ buspirone serum concentrations and ↑ busprione efficacy); *carbamazepine
(↑ carbamazepine toxicity); **chloral hydrate (↑ risk of cardiotoxicity); **chloro-
quine (↑ risk of cardiotoxicity) **chlorpromazine (↑ risk of cardiotoxicity); *cisapride (contraindicated, cardiotoxicity); **clarithromycin (↑ risk of cardiotoxicity);
**clindamycin (antagonistic antimicrobial effects and/or ↑ cardiotoxicity); *clozap-
ine (↑ clozapine serum concentrations and ↑ risk of side effects); **colchicine
(↑ colchicine serum levels and ↑ toxicity); *cyclosporine (↑ cyclosporine toxicity);
**desipramine (↑ risk of cardiotoxicity); *diazepam (↑ benzodiazepine toxicity);
*dicumarol (↑ risk of bleeding); **digoxin (↑ digoxin levels and digoxin toxicity);
*dihyrdoergotamine (contraindicated, ↑ risk of acute ergotism); **ditiazem (↑ risk
of cardiotoxicity); **disopyramide (↑ risk of cardiotoxicity); **dofetilide (↑ risk
of cardiotoxicity); **doxepin (↑ risk of cardiotoxicity); **droperidol (↑ risk of
cardiotoxicity); *estazolam (↑ estazolam toxicity); *oral contraceptives (↓ contraceptive efficacy and ↑ risk of hepatotoxicity); *fentanyl (↑ or prolonged opioid
efficacy); *flecainide (↑ risk of cardiotoxicity); **fluconazole (↑ risk of cardiotoxicity); **fluoxetine (↑ risk of cardiotoxicity); *fluvastatin (↑ risk of myopathy and
rhabdomyolysis); *foscarnet (↑ risk of cardiotoxicity); **gatifloxacin, gemifloxacin,
grepafloxacin (↑ risk of cardiotoxicity); **haloperidol (↑ risk of cardiotoxicity);
*ibutilide (↑ risk of cardiotoxicity); **imipramine (↑ risk of cardiotoxicity); **itraconazole (↑ concentrations of itraconazole); **ketoconazole (↑ serum concentrations of erythromycin and ketoconazole): *lovastatin (↑ risk of myopathy and
rhabdomyolysis); *methadone (↑ serum methadone levels); *methylprednisolone
(↑ risk of steroid adverse effects); *midazolam (↑ sedation); **moxifloxacin (↑ risk
of cardiotoxicity); *nifedipine (↑ nifedipine serum concentrations and ↑ nifedipine
toxicity); **nortriptyline (↑ risk of cardiotoxicity); *pravastatin (↑ risk of myopathy
and rhabdomyolysis); **procainimide (↑ risk of cardiotoxicity); **prochlorperazine
(↑ risk of cardiotoxicity); *quinidine (↑ risk of cardiotoxicity); *repaglinide (↑ repaglinide serum concentrations); **risperidone (↑ risk of cardiotoxicity); **sertraline

(↑ risk of serotonin syndrome); *sildenafil (↑ risk of sildenafil adverse effects); *simvastatin (↑ myopathy and rhabdomyolysis); **sotalol (↑ risk of cardiotoxicity); **sulfamethoxazole (↑ risk of cardiotoxicity); *tacrolimus (↑ tacrolimus concentration); *theophylline (↑ theophylline toxicity and ↓ erythromycin efficacy); *tramadol (↑ tramadol); *triazolam (↑ benzodiazepine toxicity); **trimethoprim (↑ risk of cardiotoxicity); valproic acid (↑ valproic acid toxicity); *venlafaxine (↑ risk of cardiotoxicity); **verapamil (↑ risk of cardiotoxicity); *warfarin (↑ risk of bleeding); **zolmitripton (↑ risk of cardiotoxicity).

Food/beverages

Alcohol may ↓ absorption of erythromycin or enhance alcohol effects. *Grapefruit juice (↑ efficacy, macrolide level and adverse effects may ↑). Food may ↓ efficacy.

Incompatible herbs/interaction effect

St. John's wort (↓ erythromycin levels).

Syringe incompatiblity

Ampicillin, heparin.

Y-site incompatibility

Ceftazidime, fluconazole.

Additive Incompatibility

Heparin, metoclopramide, vitamin B complex with C.

Laboratory considerations

May ↑ serum bilirubin, AST, ALT, and alkaline phosphatase. May cause false ↑ of urinary catecholamines.

Clinical management

PO; administer on empty stomach or 1 hour before or 2 hours after meals. May take with food to avoid gastrointestinal upset. Administer with full glass of water. Liquid preparation: Shake well. Do not crush or chew delayed-release capsules or tablets; swallow whole tablet. Monitor for ototoxicity with large dosages. Advise client to report signs of ototoxicty headache, dizziness, vertigo, ringing in the ears, nausea and vomiting, motion sickness, ataxia, and nystagmus. Monitor for signs and symptoms of hepatotoxicity, abdominal pain, nausea, vomiting, fever, leukocytosis, eosinophilia, and jaundice.

* Severity of reaction indicated by: * moderate, ** severe

furosemide

Furoside, Lasix

Classification: Loop diuretic
Therapeutic uses: Diuretic

Incompatible drugs/interaction effect

*Amikacin (↑ ototoxicity and/or nephrotoxicity); *ACE inhibitors [{alacepril, bena-zepril, captopril, cilazapril, enalapril, fosinopril, lisinopril, moexipril, quinapril, ramipril} ↑ postural hypotension first dose]; amphotericin B (↑ hypokalemia); *aspirin (↓ diruetic efficacy); *cholestyramine (↓ furosemide efficacy); *clofibrate (↑ diuretic efficacy, muscle pain and stiffness, ↑ serum transaminases and creatine phosphokinases); *colestipol (↓ furosemide efficacy); *cortisone (hypokalemia); *digoxin (↑ digoxin toxicity); **dofetilide (↑ risk cardiotoxicity); *ethacrynic acid (↑ risk ototoxicity); *fludocortisone (hypkalemia); *fosphenytoin (↓ furosemide efficacy); *gentamycin (↑ ototoxicity and nephrotoxicity, altered plasma levels of gentamycin); *hydrocortisone (hypokalemia); *lithium (↑ lithium concentration and ↑ lithium toxicity); *phenytoin (↓ furosemide efficacy); *propranolol (hypo-tension and bradycardia); *sotalol (↑ risk cardiotoxicity); *theophylline (altered theophylline levels); *NSAIDs [{aceclofenac, alclofenac, benoxaprofen, bromfenac, carprofen, celecoxib, clometacin, diclofenac, diflunisal, etodolac, etofenamate, felbinac, fenbufen, flurbiprofen, ibuprofen, indomethacin, isoxicam, ketoprofen, ketorolac, meclofenamate, meloxicam, nabumetone, naproxen, oxaprozin, oxy-phenbutazone, phenylbutazone, pipercillin (↑ hypokalemia); piroxicam, probenecid, propyphenazone, sulcrafate (↓ furosemide efficacy); sulindac, tenoxicam, tolmetin) ↓ diuretic and antihypertensive efficacy]; warfarin (↑ warfarin efficacy).

Food/beverages

Alcohol (↑ hypotension).

Incompatible herbs/interaction effect

*Ginseng (↑ risk of diuretic resistance); licorice (↑ risk of QT prolongation); *Ma huang (↓ diuretic efficacy); yohimbine (↓ diuretic efficacy).

Y-site incompatibility

Ciprofloxacin, diltiazem, dobutamine, dopamine, doxapram, doxorubicin, droperidol, epinephrine, esmolol, fenoldopam mesylate, filgrastin, fluconazole, gatifloxacin, gemcitabine, gentamycin, hydralazine, idarubicin, inamrinone, levofloxacin, metoclopramide, midazolam, milrinone, morphine, ondansetron, quinidine gluconate, tetracycline, thiopental, vecuronium, vinblastine, vincristine, vinorelbine.

Syringe incompatibility
Doxapram, doxorubicin, droperidol, metoclopramide, milrinone, vinblastine, vincristine.

Lab test interactions
May cause ↓ serum potassium, calcium, and magnesium. May ↑ BUN, serum glucose, creatinine, and uric acid levels.

Clinical management
PO; administer with food or milk to ↓ gastrointestinal irritation. Advise client to consult healthcare provider before taking any other medications or supplements. Client should wear sunscreen and protective clothing in the sun to prevent photosensitivity. Caution client not to change brands of furosemide since bioavailability varies. Monitor for signs and symptoms of dehydration, hypotension, and bradycardia. Monitor serum electrolytes. Advise client to notify healthcare provider of dizziness, numbness, muscle weakness, or cramps.

* Severity of reaction indicated by: * moderate, ** severe

gentamicin
Garamycin, IV, IM

Classification: Aminoglycoside
Therapeutic uses: Antibiotic, anti-infective

Incompatible drugs/interaction effect
*Butamide (↑ otoxicity); *cyclosporine (↑ nephrotoxicity); *ethacrynic acid (↑ ototoxicity); *furosemide (↑ serum levels of gentamycin, ↑ ototoxicity/ ↑ nephrotoxicity); *indomethacin (↑ gentamycin toxicity); **lysine (↑ nephrotoxicity); *magnesium (↑ neuromuscular weakness); *succinylcholine (enhanced neuromuscular blockade); **tacrolimus (↑ renal function impairment); **vancomycin (↑ nephrotoxicity).

Y-site incompatibility: Allopurinol, amphotericin B, ampicillin, carbenicillin, cefoperazone, cefotetan, ceftazidime, cephalothin, cepharpirin, cloxacillin, furosemide, idarubicin, mezlocillin, indomethacin, sulfamethoxazole/ trimethoprim, phenytoin, pipercillin, ticarcillin.

Clinical management: Advise client to report signs of ototoxicty headache, dizziness, vertigo, ringing in the ears, nausea and vomiting, motion sickness, ataxia, and nystagmus. Clients should immediately report any changes in urinary elimination, decreased urine output, and unusual appearance of urine. Peak and trough levels should be monitored for therapeutic levels and to avoid toxicity. Monitor BUN and creatinine serum levels for nephrotoxity.

* Severity of reaction indicated by: * moderate, ** severe

heparin
Hep-Lock, Hep-Lock U/P, Heparin Sodium, Heparin Calcium, Heparin Lock Flush

Classification: Anticoagulant
Therapeutic uses: Antithrombotic

Incompatible drugs/interaction effect
**Abciximab, **altepase, **aspirin, **cefamandole, **cefoperazone, **clopidogrel, **dextran, **moxalactam, **reviparin, (↑ risk of bleeding).

Food/beverages
Alfalfa (↓ efficacy); avocado (↓ anticoagulant effectiveness). Alcohol (↑ risk of bleeding).

Incompatible herbs/interaction effect
*Angelica, *anise, *bilberry, *black currant, *capsaicin, *cat's claw, *celery, *chamomile, *chondroitin, *clove oil, *devil's claw, *Dong Quai, *fenugreek, *feverfew, **garlic, ginger, **ginkgo, *kava, *licorice, papaya, skullcap, St. John's wort , vitamin A (↑ risk of bleeding). Coenzyme Q10 (↓ anticoagulant effectiveness).

Y-site incompatibility
Alteplase, amiodarone, amphotericin B cholesteryl sulfate, ciprofloxacin, diazepam, doxycycline, ergotamine tartrate, filgrastim, gatifloxacin, gentamycin,

haloperidol, idarubicin, levofloxacin, phenytoin, tobramycin, trifupromazine, vancomycin.

Syringe incompatibility

Amikacin, amiodarone, chlorpromazine, diazepam, doxorubicin, droperidol, erythromycin, lactobionate, gentamycin, haloperidol, kanamycin, merperidine, pentazocine, promethiazine, streptomycin, tobramycin, triflupromazine, vancomycin, warfarin.

Lab test interactions

May cause ↑ in AST and ALT levels. ↑ thyroxine levels; ↑ PT.

Clinical management

Monitor for bleeding and hemorrhage (unusual bruising, bleeding gums, nosebleed, black tarry stools, hematuria, ↓ hematocrit, hyperkalemia, peripheral neuropathy and ↓ blood pressure). Monitor CBC, aPTT, INR. Instruct client to monitor for signs of bleeding. Protect from injury, chest pain or CNS changes, painful joints, and to check with healthcare provider before taking any other medications or OTCs.

* Severity of reaction indicated by: * moderate, ** severe

hydrochlorothiazide

Chlorothiazide, HCTZ, Microzide

Classification: Thiazide diuretic
Therapeutic uses: Antihypertensive, diuretic

Incompatible drugs/interaction effect

*ACE inhibitors [{acepril, benazepril, captopril, cilazapril, enalapril, fosinopril, lisinopril, moexipril, quinalpril, ramipril} ↑ postural hypotension]; *calcitrol (↑ hypercalcemia); *calcium carbonate (milk-alkali syndrome; hypercalemia, metabolic acidosis, renal failure); *carbamazepine (hypnatremia); *choloropropramide (↓ choloropropramide efficacy); *cholestyramine (↓ hydrochlorothiazide efficacy); *colestipol (↓ hydrochlorothiazide efficacy); *corticotropin (hypokalemia); *cortisone (hypokalemia); *diazoxide (hyperglycemia); *digoxin (↑ digoxin toxicity); **dofetilide (contraindicated, ↑ risk of cardiotoxicity); *fludocortisone (hypokalemia and ↑ cardiac arrhythmias); *fluorouracil (myelosuppression); *glipizide (↓ glipizide efficacy); *glyburide (↓ glyburide efficacy); hyrdrocortisone (hypokalemia and ↑ cardiac arrhythmias); lithium (↑ serum lithium levels and lithium toxicity); methotrexate (myelosuppression); *methylprednisolone (hypokalemia and ↑ cardiac arrhythmias); *NSAIDs [{acemetacin, alclofenac, apazone, bromfenac, carprofen, celecoxib, clometacin, diclofenac, diflunisol, etodolac, etofenamate, fenbufen, fenoprofen, fentiazac, ibuprofen, indomethacin, isoxicam, ketoprofen, ketorolac, meclofenamate, meloxicam, nambutone, naproxen, oxaprozin, phenylbutazone, piroxicam, propyphenazone, sulindac, tenoxicam, tolmetin} ↓ diuretic and hypertensive efficacy]; *prednisone (hypokalemia); *propranolol (hyperglycemia and hypertriglyceridemia); **sotalol (↑ risk cardiotoxicity); **tolbutamide (↓ tolbutamide efficacy); *triamcinolone (↑ hypokalemia and cardiac arrhythmias).

Food/beverages
Peak serum levels may be decreased by food. May deplete potassium, sodium, and magnesium.

Incompatible herbs/interaction effect
Ginkgo (↑ blood pressure); licorice (↑ risk of hypoglycemia and efficacy); Ma huang (↓ hypertensive effects); yohimbine (↓ diuretic efficacy). Aloe, cascara sagrada, senna may cause ↓ potassium levels.

Lab test interactions
False increases in acetaminophen levels. May ↑ CPK, ammonia, amylase, calcium, chloride, cholesterol, glucose levels. May ↓ chloride, magnesium, potassium, sodium, tyramine, phentolamine tests, histamine tests for pheochromocytoma.

Clinical management
PO; may be administered with food or milk. Monitor periodic serum electrolytes while taking this drug. Monitor for ↓ blood pressure, weight, I&O, and signs of dehydration. Advise client of signs and symptoms of dehydration (thirst, weakness, dizziness, confusion, fainting, fever, rapid heart rate, decreased BP, hot dry skin, decreased urine output) to report to healthcare provider.

* Severity of reaction indicated by: * moderate, ** severe

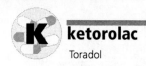

ketorolac

Toradol

Classification: Pyrroxiline carboxylic acid

Therapeutic uses: Nonsteroidal anti-inflammatory agent, nonopioid analgesic

Incompatible drugs/interaction effect

Acetaminophen (↑ risk of adverse renal reactions); *acetohexamide (↑ risk of hypoglycemia); cefotetan, cefoperazone (↑ risk of bleeding);* diuretics [{amiloride, spironolactone, triamterene (↓ diuretic effectiveness, hyperkalemia or nephrotoxicity)], azosemide, bumetanide, chlorothiazide, ethacrynic acid, furosemide, hydrochlorothiazide} ↓ diuretic and antihypertensive efficacy] ; *chloropropramide (↑ risk of hypoglycemia); *citalopram (↑ risk of bleeding); *clopidogrel (↑ risk of bleeding); *cyclosporine (↑ risk of cyclosporine toxicity); *dicumarol (↑ INR serum values and potentiation of anticoagulant effects); *dalteparin (↑ risk of bleeding); *digoxin (↑ risk of digoxin toxicity); femoxetine (↑ risk of bleeding); fluoxetine (↑ risk of bleeding); *glimepiride, *glypizide, *glyburide (↑ risk of hypoglycemia); *iron (↓ iron availability); itraconazole (↓ itraconazole efficacy); *ketoconazole (↓ ketoconazole efficacy); *levofloxacin, norfloxacin, ofloxacin (↑ risk of seizures); *lithium (↑ lithium toxicity); **metho-trexate (↑ methotrexate toxicity); **NSAIDs [{aspirin, alclofenac, alclofenal, clometacin, diclofenac, diclofenac, diflunisal, etodolac, etofenamate, felbinac, fenoprofen, ibuprofen, indomethacin, ketoprofen, meclofenamate, meloxicam, nabumetone, naproxen, oxaprozin, oxicam, phenylbutazone, piroxicam, propy-phenazone, sulinac, tolmetin} ketorolac is contraindicated in clients receiving aspirin or NSAIDs due to cummlative NSAID-related adverse effects; peptic ulcers, gastrointestinal bleeding, and/or perforation]; *paroxetine (↑ risk of bleeding); *probenecid (↑ ketorolac serum levels and toxicity);**reviparin (↑ risk of bleed-ing); *sertraline (↑ risk of bleeding); **tacrolimus (↑ tacrolimus concentration and acute renal failure); *tolazamide (↑ hypoglycemia); *tolbutamide (↑ hypo-glycemia); warfarin (↑ INR serum values and potentiation of anticoagulant effects); valproic acid (↑ risk of bleeding); *venlafaxine (↑ risk of bleeding).

Food/beverages

Avoid alcohol (↑ gastrointestinal irritation); high-fat food may delay peak time and ↓ peak concentrations.

Incompatible herbs/interaction effect

Arnica (↑ risk of bleeding); chamomile (↑ risk of bleeding); Dong Quai (↑ risk of bleeding); feverfew (↑ risk of gastropathy, ↑ risk of bleeding, and nephropathy); garlic (↑ risk of bleeding); ginger (↑ risk of bleeding); ginkgo (↑ risk of bleeding); Ma huang (↑ gastric ulcers).

Y-site incompatibility
Azithromycin, fenoldopam.

Syringe incompatibility
Diazepam, haloperidol, hydroxyzine, meperidine, morphine, prochlorperazine, promethazine, remifentanil, sufentanil.

Lab test interactions
May cause ↑ AST, ALT, BUN, serum creatinine, potassium concentrations, and may prolong bleeding time for 24–48 hours after discontinuation.

Clinical management
Avoid concurrent use with other NSAIDs. PO; administer with food or milk to ↓ gastrointestinal distress. Ketorolac will be initially started either IM or IV before oral therapy. Teach client to avoid using alcohol, other NSAIDs, acetaminophen, or other medications without checking with healthcare provider. Instruct client to report signs of gastrointestinal bleeding (abdominal pain, blood in stool or urine, ringing in the ears, respiratory difficulty, unusual swelling of extremities, flulike muscle aches and pain, including chills and fever, chest pain, or palpitations). Instruct client to report signs of gastrointestinal bleeding (abdominal pain, blood in stool or urine) or ringing in ears to healthcare providers.

* Severity of reaction indicated by: * moderate, ** severe

lansoprazole
Prevacid, Prevacid SoluTab

Classification: Proton pump inhibitor
Therapeutic uses: Antiulcer agent

Incompatible drugs/interaction effect
*Aluminum carbonate, *aluminum hydroxide, *aluminum phosphate (↓ lansoprazole availability); *ampicillin (↓ ampicillin efficacy); *calcium carbonate (↓ lansoprazole availability); *dicumarol (↑ INR serum values and potentiation of anticoagulant

effects); digoxin (↑ risk of digoxin toxicity); *itraconazole (↓ itraconazole efficacy); ketoconazole (↓ ketoconazole efficacy); *magnesium carbonate (↓ lansoprazole availability); *magnesium oxide (↓ lansoprazole availability); protease inhibitors [{atazanavir and indinavir} ↓ absorption]; sulcrafate (↓ lansoprazole availability); tacrolimus (↑ tacrolimus concentration); **warfarin (↑ INR serum values and potentiation of anticoagulant effects).

Food/beverages
Cranberry (↓ efficacy); taken with food (↓ lansoprazole concentrations).

Incompatible herbs/interaction effect
St. John's wort (↓ efficacy).

Site incompatibility
Do not mix with other IV solutions or drugs.

Syringe incompatibility
Do not mix with other IV solutions or drugs.

Lab test interactions
May cause abnormal AST, ALT, alkaline phosphatase, LDH, bilirubin, ↑ serum creatinine, ↑ gastrin levels, abnormal A/G ratio, hyperlipidemia, ↑ or ↓ electrolyte levels, ↑ or ↓ cholesterol. May interfere with RBC, WBC, and platelet levels.

Clinical management
Administer without food or before meals. Capsules may be opened and sprinkled on top 1 Tbsp of food and swallowed immediately. Do not crush or chew capsule contents. Oral disintegrating tablet may be placed on tongue and allowed to dissolve or swallowed with or without water. For NG/TP/GT administration, capsules may be opened and mixed with 40 mL of juice, injected, then tube flushed. Reconstitute IV preparation 30 mg vial with 5 mL of sterile water. Other dilutions will cause precipitation.

* **Severity of reaction indicated by: * moderate, ** severe**

levothyroxine

Levothroid, Levoxyl, Novothyrox, Synthroid, T 4, Unithroid, Liothyronine (Cytomel, l-triiodothyronine, T 3 , Triostat), Liotrix, (T 3/ T 4, Thyrolar), Thyroid (Armour thyroid, Thyrar, Thyroid Strong, Westhroid)

Classification: Thyroid hormone
Therapeutic uses: Thyroid replacement

Incompatible drugs/interaction effect

*Acenocoumarol (↑ risk of bleeding); *aluminum carbonate, *aluminum hydroxide, *aluminum phosphate (↓ levothyroxine efficacy); adrenergics (↑ cardiovascular effects), beta-blockers (↓ efficacy); bile acid sequestrants (↓ absorption with oral preparations; ↓ efficacy), *calcium carbonate (↓ levothyroxine absorption); *cholestyramine (↓ levothyroxine efficacy); dicumarol (↑ risk of bleeding); *estrogen therapy [{conjugated estrogens, esterified estrogens, estradiol, estrone, estropipate, ethinyl estradiol}↑ need for thyroid replacement; ↓ efficacy], *fosphenytoin (↓ levothyroxine efficacy); insulin or oral hypoglycemics (↑ need for replacement); *iron salts [{ferrous fumarate, ferrous gluconate, ferrous sulfate, iron polysaccharide}↓ efficacy and hypothyroidism]; *magnesium carbonate, magnesium hydroxide, magnesium oxide (↓ levothyroxine efficacy); *phenindione (↑ risk of bleeding); *phenytoin (↓ levothyroxine efficacy); *protease inhibitors [{lopinavir, ritonavir} ↓ levothyroxine efficacy]; rifampin (↓ levothyroxine efficacy).

Food/beverages

*Kelp (↑ risk of hypo- or hyperthyroidism, altered thyroid dosage requirements and inaccurate thyroid function tests). Soybean (↓ levothyroxine efficacy). Warfarin (↑ risk of bleeding). Soybean flour (infant formula), cottonseed meal, walnuts, and dietary fiber may ↓ absorption of levothryoxine from gastrointestinal tract.

Y-site incompatibility

Do not mix with other IV solutions or drugs.

Syringe incompatibility

Do not mix with other IV solutions or drugs.

Clinical management

Administer on an empty stomach at least 30 minutes before food. PO; advise client that aluminum, magnesium, calcium carbonate, cholestyramine, colestipol, iron, kayexalate, simethicone, or sulcralfate may decrease T4 absorption; separate dose from levothyroxine by at least 4 hours. Instruct client not to discontinue medication without consulting with healthcare provider first. Advise client not to take levothyroxine with other medications without consulting healthcare provider. Inform client to take levoxyl tablets with full glass of water and swallow immediately to avoid tablets swelling and becoming choking hazard. Client should notify healthcare provider immediately for signs of toxicity: chest pain, palpitations, nervousness, tachycardia, excessive sweating.

* Severity of reaction indicated by: * moderate, ** severe

lithium

Eskalith, Eskalith-CR, Lithobid, Lithonate, Lithotabs

Classification: CNS agent, antimanic agent
Therapeutic uses: Mood stabilizer

Incompatible drugs/interaction effect

*Acetazolamide (↓ lithium efficacy or ↑ serum lithium level and risk for toxicity); *ACE inhibitors [{alacepril, benazepril, captopril, enalaprilat, enalapril maleate, fosinopril, lisinopril} ↑ lithium toxicity and nephrotoxicity]; **angiotensin II inhibitors {candesartan cilexetil, losartan} ↑ risk of toxicity]; *amiloride, *bumetanide, *azosemide, *furosemide (↑ serum lithium levels and lithium toxicity); calcitonin (↓ serum lithium level and ↓ efficacy); *carbamazepine (↑ neurotoxicity); *celecoxib (↑ serum lithium levels and risk of toxicity); **chlorothiazide (↑ serum lithium levels and toxicity); **chloropromazine (↑ extrapyramidal symptoms, weakness, encephalopathy, and brain damage); **clozapine (↑ extrapyramidal symptoms, weakness, encephalopathy, and brain damage); diltiazem (↑ neurotoxicity, psychosis); **ethcrynic acid (↑ serum lithium level and toxicity); femoxetine (↑ serum lithium level and ↑ risk of SSRI related serotonin syndrome); *filgrastim (↑ WBC); fluoxetine (↑ serum lithium level and ↑ risk of SSRI related serotonin syndrome); haloperidol (↑ extrapyramidal symptoms, weakness, encephalopathy, and brain damage); ** hydrochlorothiazide (↑ serum lithium levels and risk of toxicity); insulin (↑ hypoglycemia or hyperglycemia); insulin glargine (↑ hypoglycemia or hyperglycemia); *methyldopa (↑ risk of lithium toxicity); *paroxetine (↑ serum lithium level and ↑ risk of SSRI related serotonin syndrome); **phenelzine (↑ risk of malignant hyperpyrexia); *phenylbutazone (↑ risk of lithium toxicity); *potassium iodide (↑ hypothyroid effect); **prochorperazine (↑ extrapyramidal

symptoms, weakness, encephalopathy, and brain damage); **promazine
(↑ extrapyramidal symptoms, weakness, encephalopathy, and brain damage);
**prochlorperazine (↑ extrapyramidal symptoms, weakness, encephalopathy, and
brain damage); NSAIDs [{alclofenac, diclofenac, diflunisal, etodolac, etofenamate,
fenoprofen, ibuprofen, indomethacin, ketoprofen, ketorolac, meclofenamate,
meloxicam, naproxen} ↑ lithium toxicity]; probenecid (↑ risk of lithium toxicity).

Food/beverages

↑ lithium serum concentrations with food. Limit caffeine. Low sodium levels may
cause lithium toxicity. High sodium levels may decrease lithium efficacy; psyllium
(↓ serum lithium levels).

Incompatible herbs/interaction effect

Guarana (↑ serum lithium level).

Lab test interactions

May cause falsely ↑ sodium levels.

Clinical management

Administer with food or milk to decrease gastrointestinal upset. Instruct client
not to overexert or exercise in hot weather. Report fever, vomiting, and diarrhea,
which cause sodium depletion, to healthcare provider. Monitor lithium levels
every two months during maintenance therapy. Review with client signs and
symptoms of toxicity to report to healthcare provider (vomiting, diarrhea, slurred
speech, disturbance in motor coordination, drowsiness, muscle weakness, and
twitching). Instruct client to drink 2 L–3 L of water daily. Consult with client
about sodium in diet. Caution client not to stop drug abruptly.

* Severity of reaction indicated by: * moderate, ** severe

methocarbamol
Carbacot, Robaxin

Classification: Skeletal muscle relaxant
Therapeutic uses: Muscle relaxant, skeletal

Incompatible drugs/interaction effect
*Alcohol, *antihistamines, **benzodiazepines [{alprazolam, clonezepam, diazepam, estazolam, flurazepam, lorazepam, midazolam, oxazepam, **opioid analgesics [{hydrocodone, hydromorphone, meperidine, morphine, oxycodone, oxymorphone, proxyphene}]; **sedative/hypnotics [{afentanil, fentanyl, levorphanol, pentobarbitol, sufentanil}]; **carisoprodol, **chloral hydrate, **chlordiazepoxide, **clorazepate, **codeine, **dantrolene, **phenobarbital.

Food/beverages
Alcohol ↑ CNS depression.

Incompatible herbs/interaction effect
↑ CNS depression with kava, valerian, skullcap, chamomile, or hops.

Lab test interactions
May cause falsely elevated urinary 5-hydroxyindoleacetic acid (5-HIAA) and vanillylmandelic acid (VMA) determinations.

Clinical management
May be administered with food to prevent gastrointestinal upset. Tablet may be crushed and mixed with water for NG/TP/GT tubes. Do not administer subcutaneously. Monitor IV site for thrombophlebitis. Injection is hypertonic. Instruct client not combine with other CNS depressants and to check with healthcare provider before adding any medications. Educate client that urine may become dark to brown or green on standing. WBCs should be monitored during long-term use.

* Severity of reaction indicated by: * moderate, ** severe

methylprednisolone

Depo-Medrol, Medrol, Solu-Medrol

Classification: Systemic corticosteroid
Therapeutic uses: Anti-inflammatory, immunosuppressant

Incompatible drugs/interaction effect

*Acenocoumarol (↑ risk of bleeding and ↓ anticoagulant efficacy); *amphotericin B
(↑ hypokalemia); *aspirin (↑ risk of gastrointestinal ulcers and ↓ therapeutic aspirin
levels); *balofloxacin, cinoxacin, ciprofloxacin, clinafloxacin, enoxacin, *fleroxacin,
gemifloxacin, grepafloxacin, levofloxacin, lomefloxacin, moxifloxacin, norfloxacin,
ofloxacin, trovafloxacin (↑ risk of tendon rupture); *bupropion (contraindicated,
↑ seizure); *carbamazepine (↓ methylprednisolone efficacy); *clarithromycin
(↑ risk steroid side effects); *cyclosporine (cyclosporine toxicity and steroid excess);
*dalfopristine (↑ methylprednisolone side effects); *dicumarol (↑ risk of bleeding or
↓ anticoagulant effects); *diltiazem (↑ methylprednisolone serum concentrations);
*erythromycin (↑ steroid side effects); *fosphenytoin (↓ methylprednisolone efficacy);
*hydrochlorothiazide (↑ hypokalemia and ↑ cardiac arrhythmias); itraconazole, keta-
conazole (↑ serum corticosteroid concentrations and ↑ risk of corticosteroid side
effects); phenindione (↑ risk of bleeding and ↓ anticoagulant effects); *phenobarbital
(↓ methylprednisolone efficacy); *phenytoin (↓ methylprednisolone efficacy); *primi-
done (↓ methylprednisolone efficacy); *quinupristine (↑ risk of methylprednisolone
side effects); *rifampin (↓ methylprednisolone efficacy); *tacrolimus (↑ tacrolimus
concentrations); *warfarin (↑ risk of bleeding or ↓ anticoagulant efficacy).

Food/beverages

Avoid alcohol (↑ gastrointestinal irritation); interferes with calcium absorption.

Incompatible herbs/interaction effect

*Echinacea (↓ efficacy corticosteroids); *licorice (↑ corticosteroid side effects); *Ma
huang (↓ corticoidsteroid efficacy); St. John's wort (↓ methylprednisolone levels).

Y-site incompatibility

Allopurinol, amphotericin B cholesteryl sulfate, cefepime, ciprofloxacin, doxorubicin, filgrastim, furosemide, odansetron, propofol, sargramostim, vinorelbine.

Syringe incompatibility

Doxapram.

Incompatible IV fluids

D 5 ¹/₂ NS.

Lab test interactions

False ↑ digoxin levels.

Clinical management:

Administer PO with food to decrease gastrointestinal upset and irritation. May cause loss of glycemic control in diabetics. Monitor glucose and hemoglobin A1C. Monitor for hypokalemia. Advise client not to stop medication abruptly and to take all doses as instructed. Client should check with healthcare provider before taking additional medications with this drug. CBC, AST, ALT, serum electrolytes, BUN, creatinine, and total cholesterol should be monitored periodically. Client should report abdominal pain, blood in stool, cramping in legs, headache, dizziness, increased blood pressure, unusual bleeding or increased bruising, infections and colds that do not resolve, wounds that do not heal, and mood disturbances that interfere with daily activities to healthcare provider.

* Severity of reaction indicated by: * moderate, ** severe

metronidazole

Flagyl, Flagyl ER, Fagyl

Classification: Miscellaneous

Therapeutic uses: Antibiotic, anti-infective, antiprotozoal, antiulcer, amebicide

Incompatible drugs/interaction effect

**Amiodarone (↑ risk of cardiac toxicity); **amprenavir (↑ risk of propylene glycol toxicity); *carbamazepine (↑ carbamazepine serum concentrations and potential carbamazepine toxicity); *cholestyramine (↓ metronidazole efficacy); cimetidine (may ↑ metronidazole levels); *cyclosporine (↑ cyclosporine toxicity); *dicumarol (↑ risk of bleeding); **dihydroergotamine (↑ risk of ergotism; nausea, vomiting, and vasospastic ischemia); **disulfiram (↑ CNS toxicity); **ergotamine (↑ risk of ergotism; nausea, vomiting, and vasospastic ischemia); **fluorouracil (↑ fluorouracil toxicity); *fosphenytoin (↑ risk of phenytoin toxicity or ↓ metronidazole serum levels); *lithium (↑ serum lithium levels and lithium toxicity); *phenytoin (↑ risk of phenytoin toxicity or ↓ metronidazole serum levels); *tacrolimus (↑ tacrolimus levels and ↑ risk tacrolimus toxicity); *warfarin (↑ risk bleeding).

Food/beverages

Avoid alcohol for at least 24 hours after administration (causes disulfiram-type adverse reaction (nausea, vomiting, headache, sweating, tachycardia). Food lowers and delays peak serum level, but total drug absorption is not affected.

Incompatible herbs/interaction effect

Valerian (vomiting).

Y-site incompatibility

Discontinue primary IV during infusion as recommended by manufacturer. Amphotericin B cholesteryl sulfate, aztreonam, filgrastim.

Syringe incompatibility

Do not mix with other medications.

Incompatible IV fluids

N/A

Lab test interactions

May alter results of AST, ALT, glucose, LDH, and triglyceride tests.

Clinical management

PO; administer on empty stomach. May take with food or milk to prevent gastrointestinal upset. Extended release should be taken 1 hour before food or 2 hours after. Advise client to perform frequent mouth care for metallic taste and dry mouth. May cause urine to turn dark.

* Severity of reaction indicated by: * moderate, ** severe

meperidine

Demerol, Meperitab, Pethidine

Classification: Opioid agonists
Therapeutic uses: Opioid analgesics

Incompatible drugs/interaction effect

*Acetophenazine (↑ CNS and respiratory depression); *acyclovir (↑ CNS stimulation and excitation); **alfentanil (↑ respiratory depression); **butorphanol (causes withdrawal symptoms, abdominal cramps, nausea, vomiting, lacrimation,

anxiety, restlessness, fever); **benzodiazepines [{alprazolam, diazepam, clonazepam, estazolam, lorazepam, midazolam, oxazepam, temazepam, triazolam}
↑ respiratory depression]; **carisoprodol (↑ respiratory depression); **chloral
hydrate (↑ respiratory depression); **chlordiazepoxide (↑ respiratory depression);
**chlorpromazine (↑ CNS and respiratory depression); **cimetidine (meperidine
toxicity, ↑ respiratory depression, and hypotension); **clorazepate (↑ respiratory
depression); **codeine (↑ respiratory depression); **dantrolene (↑ respiratory
depression) **fentanyl (↑ respiratory depression); **fluphenazine (↑ CNS and respiratory depression); **fosphenytoin (↓ meperidine efficacy); **hydrocodone (↑ respiratory depression); **hydromorphone (↑ respiratory depression); **isoniazid
(↑ hypotension and CNS depression, **levophanol (↑ respiratory depression);
**MAOIs (procarbazine contraindicated, causes cardiac instability, hyperpyrexia,
and coma); **methocarbamol (↑ respiratory depression); **oxycodone (↑ respiratory depression); **phenobarbital (↑ respiratory depression); **phenytoin (↓ meperidine efficacy); **prochlorperazine, promazine, promethazine (↑ CNS and respiratory
depression); **proxyphene (↑ respiratory depression); ritonavir (↑ CNS stimulation and excitation); sufentanil (↑ respiratory depression).

Food/beverages
Ethanol (↑ sedation).

Incompatible herbs/interaction effect
St. John's wort (↑ sedation), kava (↑ CNS depression), gotu kola (↑ CNS depression), valerian (↑ CNS depression).

Y-site incompatibility
Allopurinol, anphotericin B cholesteryl sulfate, cefepime, cefoperazone, doxorubicin, furosemide, heparin, idarubicin, imipenem/cilastatin, minocycline, mezlocillin, morphine, phenobarbital, phenytoin, tetracycline.

Syringe incompatibility
Heparin, pentobarbital.

Lab test interactions
May ↑ serum amylase and lipase.

Clinical management
PO; may be administered with food or milk to decrease gastrointestinal upset.
Monitor for respiratory depression, bradycardia, and hypotension. Instruct client
not to use alcohol, other CNS depressants, or other drugs without consulting

healthcare provider. Repeated SQ doses may cause local irritation. IV: Administer slowly over at least 5 min. Rapid administration is contraindicated and can lead to respiratory depression, hypotension, and circulatory collapse.

* Severity of reaction indicated by: * moderate, ** severe

morphine

Astramorph, Astramorph PF, Avinza, Duramorph, Kadian, Infumorph, MSIR, Roxanol, MS Contin, Oramorph SR.

Classification: Opioid analgesic
Therapeutic uses: Opioid agonist

Incompatible drugs/interaction effect

**Alfentanil (↑ respiratory depression); **alprazolam (↑ respiratory depression); **antihistamines (↑ CNS and respiratory depression); *buprenorphine (↓ efficacy and analgesia); *butorphanol (↓ efficacy and analgesia); **carisoprodol (↑ respiratory depression); **chloral hydrate (↑ respiratory depression); **chlordiazepoxide (↑ respiratory depression); **chlorpromazine (↑ respiratory depression); **clomipramine (↑ respiratory depression); **cimetidine (morphine toxicity; CNS depression and ↑ respiratory depression; **clonazepam (↑ respiratory depression); codeine (↑ respiratory depression); *cyclosporine (↑ neurotoxicity and decrease neuro function); **dantrolene (↑ respiratory depression); **diazepam (↑ respiratory depression); *esmolol (esmolol toxicity, bradycardia, hypotension); **estazolam (↑ respiratory depression); **fentanyl (↑ respiratory depression); flurazepam (↑ respiratory depression); *gabapentin (↑ respiratory depression); hydrocodone (↑ respiratory depression); hydromorphone (↑ respiratory depression); levophanol (↑ respiratory depression); lorazepam (↑ respiratory depression); **meperidine (↑ respiratory depression); *metformin (↑ metformin plasma concentration); **methocarbamol (↑ respiratory depression); **midazolam (↑ respiratory depression); *nalbuphine (↓ efficacy and analgesia); **oxazepam (↑ respiratory depression); **oxycodone (↑ respiratory depression); **oxymorphone (↑ respiratory depression); **pentazocine [causes withdrawal symptoms {abdominal cramps, nausea, vomiting, rhinorrhea, anxiety, restlessness, fever, ↓ efficacy and analgesia]; **pentobarbital (↑ respiratory depression); **perhenazine (↑ CNS and respiratory depression); **phenelzine (contraindicated); **phenobarbital (↑ respiratory depression); **procarbazine (↑ hypotension, CNS and respiratory depression); **promazine (↑ CNS and respiratory depression); **promethazine (↑ CNS and respiratory depression); **propoxyphene (↑ respiratory depression); rifampin

↓ morphine efficacy); sufentanil (↑ respiratory depression); triazolam (↑ respiratory depression); **tricyclic antidepressants (↑ CNS and respiratory depression).

Food/beverages

Alcohol ↑ risk of CNS depression, hypotension, sedation, coma.

Incompatible herbs/interaction effect

Chamomile (↑ CNS depression); kava (↑ CNS depression); ginseng (↓ opioid efficacy); St. John's wort (↑ sedation); valerian (↑ CNS depression); yohimbine (↑ analgesic and adverse effects of morphine).

Y-site incompatibility

Amphotericin B cholesteryl sulfate, azithromycin, cefepime, doxorubicin, minocycline, phenytoin, sargramostim, tetracycline.

Syringe incompatibility

Meperidine, chlorpromazine, haloperidol, heparin, pentobarbital, prochlorperazine edisylate, promethazine, thiopental.

Lab test interactions

May ↑ serum amylase and lipase levels. False-positive urine glucose readings may occur with Benedict's solution.

Clinical management

May be taken with food and water to prevent gastrointestinal upset. Monitor for respiratory depression; respirations ≤10; stimulate client to avoid hypoventilation. Monitor level of consciousness, blood pressure, and pulse for depression. Monitor for ↓ bowel sounds, constipation, and paralytic ileus. Teach client to avoid combining with other CNS depressants including alcohol and to check with healthcare provider before taking any other drug combinations. Remind client to avoid sudden postural changes to prevent orthostatic hypotension. Instruct client to ↑ fiber and fluids. Do not crush, chew, or dissolve extended-release forms, as it could result in overdose. Kadian and Avinza capsules may be opened and sprinkled in 10 mL of water and then flushed through enteral feeding tubes. Do not administer IV morphine sulfate too rapidly, as it may lead to respiratory depression, hypotension, and circulatory collapse.

* Severity of reaction indicated by: * moderate, ** severe

phenytoin

Dilantin, Diphenylhydantoin, DPH, Phenytek

Classification: Hydantoin

Therapeutic uses: Antiarrhythmic (class 1 B), anticonvulsant

Incompatible drugs/interaction effect

*Acetaminophen (↓ acetaminophen efficacy and ↑ risk of hepatotoxicity); *acetazolamide (↑ risk of osteomalacia); *acyclovir (↓ phenytoin concentrations and ↑ risk of seizure activity); *amiodarone (↑ risk of phenytoin toxicity); *amitriptyline (↑ risk of phenytoin toxicity); antacids (may ↓ absorption of oral phenytoin); *aspirin (↓ phenytoin concentrations); *atorvastatin (↓ atorvastatin efficacy); *azithromycin (↑ serum phenytoin levels); *betamethasone (↓ efficacy); *bupropion (↓ brupropion efficacy); * carbamazepine (↑ phenytoin concentration and ↓ carbamazepine concentrations); *chloramphenicol (↑ risk of phenytoin toxicity); *chlorodiazepoxide (alterations in serum phenytoin concentrations); *chlorpheniramine (↑ phenytoin toxicity); *chlorpromazine (↑ or ↓ phenytoin levels and ↓ phenothiazine levels); *cimetidine (↑ risk phenytoin toxicity); * ciprofloxacin (↑ or ↓ phenytoin levels); *clarithromycin (↑ phenytoin toxicity); *clomipramine (↑ risk phenytoin toxicity); *clopidogrel (↑ risk phenytoin toxicity); *clozapine (↓ clozapine levels with worsening psychosis); *cortisone (↓ cortisone efficacy); *cyclosporine (↓ cyclosporine serum level and ↑ risk organ rejection); despiramine (↑ risk of phenytoin toxicity); *dexamethasone (↓ dexamethasone efficacy); *diazepam (alterations in phenytoin levels); *diazoxide (↓ phenytoin efficacy); *dicumarol (↑ risk of bleeding, ↓ anticoagulant efficacy and/or phenytoin toxicity); *diltiazem (↑ risk of phenytoin toxicity); *disopyramide (↓ disopyramide efficacy); *disulfiram (↑ risk of phenytoin toxicity); *dopamine (↑ hypotension and/or cardiac arrest); *doxepin (↑ risk of phenytoin toxicity); *doxorubicin (↓ phenytoin efficacy); *doxycycline (↓ doxycycline efficacy); *ethosuximide (↓ ethosuximide concentrations); *felbamate (↑ risk of phenytoin toxicity); *fentanyl (↓ plasma concentrations of fentanyl); *fluconazole (↑ risk of phenytoin toxicity); *fludrocortisone (↓ fludrocortisone levels); *fluorouracil (↑ serum phenytoin levels and phenytoin toxicity); *fluoxetine (↑ risk of phenytoin toxicity); *folic acid (↓ phenytoin efficacy); *furosemide (↓ furosemide efficacy); *hyrdorcortisone (↓ hydrocortisone efficacy); *ibuprofen (↑ risk of phenytoin toxicity); *imipramine (↑ risk of phenytoin toxicity); isoniazid (↑ risk of phenytoin toxicity); *itraconazole (↓ serum itraconazole); ketoconazole (altered metabolism ketoconazole and phenytoin); * lamotrigine (↓ lamotrigine efficacy); *levodopa (↓ levodopa efficacy); *levothyroxine (↓ levothyroxine efficacy); *lidocaine (↑ cardiac depression; ↓ lidocaine concentrations); *meperidine (↓ meperidine efficacy); **methotrexate (↓ phenytoin efficacy and risk of methotrexate toxicity); *methylphenidate (↑ phenytoin concentrations); *methylprednisone (↓ methyl-prednisone efficacy); *metronidazole (↑ risk of phenytoin toxicity); *miconazole (↑ risk miconazole toxicity); *midazolam (↓ midazolam efficacy); *oral contraceptives (↓ contraceptive efficacy); *protease inhibitiors [{amprenavir (↓ amprevnavir efficacy), darunavir (↓ darunavir concentration and ↓ efficacy), fosamprenavir (↓ amprenavir serum concentrations and ↓ fosamprenavir efficacy), indinavir (↓ indinavir concentrations), lopinavir (↓ lopinavir efficacy), nelfinavir (↓ nelfinavir efficacy), zidovudine (↑ zidovudine concentrations)]; *nifedipine (↑ risk of phenytoin toxicity); *nortriptyline (↑ risk of phenytoin toxicity); *omeprazole (↑ risk of phenytoin toxicity); *oxcarbazepine (↑ risk of phenytoin toxicity); *paroxetine (↓ phenytoin efficacy); *perphenazine (↑ or ↓ phenytoin levels or ↓ perphenazine levels); reserpine (↓ serum phenytoin levels); sulcrafate (↓ phenytoin absorption); *ticlopidine (↑ risk of phenytoin toxicity); *tolbutamide (↑ risk of phenytoin toxicity); *trazodone (↑ serum phenytoin concentrations and ↑ risk of phenytoin toxicity); *triamcinolone (↓ triamcinolone efficacy); *trimethoprim (↑ risk of phenytoin toxicity); *valproic acid (altered valproate levels and altered phenytoin levels); *verapamil (↓ verapamil efficacy); *warfarin (↑ risk of bleeding); zidovudine (↑ serum phenytoin level).

Food/beverages
Alcohol inhibits metabolism of phenytoin and ↑ sedation. Serum phenytoin levels may be altered if taken with food.

Incompatible herbs/interaction effect
Kava (↑ CNS depression); ginkgo biloba (↓ anticonvulsant efficacy); gotu kola (↑ CNS depression); St. John's wort (↓ phenytoin efficacy), valerian (↑ CNS depression).

Y-site incompatibility
Amikacin, ciprofloxacin, diltiazem, dobutamine, enalaprilat, gatifloxacin, heparin, hydromorphone, lidocaine, linezolid, potassium chloride, sufentanil, TPN, vitamin B and C complex.

Syringe incompatibility
Do not mix with other solutions or medications, especially dextrose, which will cause precipitate to form.

Incompatible IV fluids
D5NS, D5W, fat emulsion 10%, 1/2NS.

Lab test interactions

May cause ↑ serum alkaline phosphatase, GTT, and glucose levels.

Clinical management

Administer after meals to prevent gastrointestinal upset. Shake oral suspensions well before administration. Capsules may be opened and sprinkled on food or fluids, but advise client to swallow liquid first to avoid direct contact on mucous membranes. Follow with full glass of water, milk, or food. Chewable phenytoin tab should not be interchanged with capsules because they are not bioequivalent. Do not confuse once a day extended-release forms with twice a day capsules—may result in overdose and toxicity. PO form should not be stopped abruptly, as it can lead to status epilepticus. Advise client to check with healthcare provider before taking any other medications or supplements. Do not refrigerate IV form or may cause precipitate. Avoid rapid IV administration, which may result in severe hypotension, cardiovascular collapse, or CNS depression. Enteral nutrition, serum phenytoin levels are decreased. Hold tube feedings 2 hours before and 2 hours after administration. May decrease calcium, folic acid, and vitamin D levels. Monitor diabetics for loss of glycemic control. Advise client may cause drowsiness, overgrowth of gums (gingival hyperplasia), visual disturbances (blurred or double vision), and loss of appetite. Client should report unusual bleeding or increased bruising to healthcare provider.

* Severity of reaction indicated by: * moderate, ** severe

prednisone

Cordrol, Deltasone, Liquid Pred, Meticorten, Orasone, Panasol-S, Pred-Pak, Prednicen-M, Prednicot, Prednisone Intensol, Sterapred DS, Sterapred

Classification: Corticosteroid, glucocorticoid
Therapeutic uses: Antiasthmatic, systemtic corticosteroid

Incompatible drugs/interaction effect

Antacids (↓ absorption); *amphotericin B Lipsome (↑ risk hypokalemia); *erythromycin (↑ blood levels of erythromycin and efficacy); *quinolones [{balofloxacin, ciprofloxacin, cinoxacin, enoxacin, fleroxacin, **gatifloxacin (↑ risk of ↑ blood glucose and hyperglycemia), gemifloxacin, grepafloxacin, levofloxacin, moxifloxacin, norfloxacin, ofloxacin} ↑ risk for tendon rupture]; bupropion (↓ seizure threshold); *carbamazepine (↓ prednisone effectiveness); *clarithromyin (↑ risk of psychotic symptoms); **cyclosporine (↑ risk for cyclosporine toxicity); insulin (may ↑ requirements); live vaccines (↑ risk of adverse side effects);* oral contraceptives (↑ risk of corticosteroid side effects); *fluconazole (↑ efficacy); *fosphenytoin (↓ efficacy); *hydrochlorothiazide (↑ hypokalemia and cardiac arrhythmias); isoniazid (↓ isoniazid efficacy); *itraconazole (↑ corticosteroid plasma levels and ↑ risk of corticosteroid side effects); *ketoconazole (↑ risk of corticosteroid side effects); *montelukast (severe peripheral edema); oral hypoglycemic agents (may ↑ requirements); NSAIDs (↑ risk of adverse gastrointestinal side effects); phenobarbital (↓ efficacy); phenytoin (↓ efficacy); piperacillin (↑ risk of hypokalemia); rifampin (↓ efficacy); ritonavir (↑ prednisone serum concentrations); ticarcillin (↑ risk of hypokalemia).

Incompatible herbs/interaction effect
Alfalfa (↓ efficacy); echinacea (↓ efficacy); licorice (↑ risk of corticosteroid adverse effects); ma huang (↓ efficacy corticosteroids); St. John's wort (↓ efficacy).

Lab test interactions
May ↑ serum cholesterol; ↓ serum levels of T3 and T4; ↓ uptake of thyroid hormone; cause false-negative result for nitroblue-tetrazolium test for systemic bacterial infection; suppresses skin test reactions. Digoxin (false increase in digoxin levels).

Clinical management
PO; administer after meals or with food or milk; increase dietary intake of pyridoxine, vitamin C, vitamin D, folate, calcium, and phosphorus. Do not stop abruptly. Taper after long-term use. Clients should eat a diet high in protein and calcium, low in sodium and carbohydrates. Client should report abdominal pain, blood in stool, cramping in legs, headache, dizziness, increased blood pressure, unusual bleeding or increased bruising, infections and colds that do not resolve, wounds that do not heal, and mood disturbances that interfere with daily activities to healthcare provider.

* Severity of reaction indicated by: * moderate, ** severe

promethazine
Pentazine, Phenadoz, Phenergan, Promacot, Promethegan, Promet, Prorex.

Classification: Phenothiazine, H1 blocker, histamine H1 antagonist
Therapeutic uses: Anti-emetic, antihistamine, sedative/hypnotics

Incompatible drugs/interaction effect
Alcohol, antihistamines, **cisapride (cardiotoxicity); opioid analgesics [{*meperi-dine, **methadone, **morphine, **oxycodone}; **fentanyl (↑ CNS depression

and respiratory depression); CNS depressants and other sedative/hypnotics; additive effect (↑ CNS depression and respiratory depression). Antihistamines, antidepressants, atropine, haloperidol, other phenothiazines, quinidine and disopyramide (↑ anticholinergic effects). Lithium (↑ extrapyramidal symptoms, encephalopathy, and brain damage); MAOIs (↑ sedation and anticholinergic effects). *Anticholinergics [{atopine, belladonna, benzotropine, biperiden, dicyclomine, hyoscyamine, oxybutynin, propantheline, scopolamine} ↓ phenothiazine effects]. *phenobarbital (↓ promethazine efficacy); *phenytoin (↑ ↓ phenytoin level and ↓ phenothiazine levels); phenylalanine (↑ risk of tardive dyskinesia); (**quinolones [(gatifloxacin, levofloxacin, moxifloxacin, sparfloxacin) {↑ risk of life-threatening arrhythmias}]; tramadol (↑ risk of seizures); trazodone (↑ seizures).

Food/beverages
Avoid alcohol (↑ CNS depression).

Incompatible herbs/interaction effect
Gotu kola, kava, St. John's wort, valerian (may ↑ CNS depression).

Y-site incompatibility
Aldesleukin, amphotericin B cholesteryl, cefepime, cefoperazone, cefotetan, doxorubicin liposome, foscarnet, methotrexate, piperacillin/tazobactam.

Syringe incompatibility
Heparin, ketorolac, pentobarbital, thiopental.

Lab test interactions
May cause false-positive or false-negative pregnancy tests, ↑ serum glucose, or false-negative allergen skin tests.

Clinical management
PO; take with food or milk. IV: IV administration may cause severe tissue damage. Dilute solutions are recommended. Administer in running IV port farthest from client's vein over 10–15 minutes. Discontinue immediately if burning or pain occurs with administration. Rapid IV administration may cause hypotension. Monitor CBC for blood dyscrasias with long-term use. Advise client to check with healthcare provider before taking any other medications or supplements. Client should notify healthcare provider for onset of extrapyramidal side effects [akathisia (restlessness), dystonia (muscle spasms and uncoordinated motion),

pseudoparkinsionism (masklike facial expression, rigidity, tremors, drooling, shuffling gait, and dysphagia)]. Elderly may exhibit acute confusion, delirium.

* Severity of reaction indicated by: * moderate, ** severe

simvastatin
Zocar

Classification: HMG-CoA Reductase Inhibitor, statin
Therapeutic uses: Lipid lowering agent

Incompatible drugs/interaction effect
[{**Amiodarone, **ciprofibrate, **clarithromycin, **clofibrate, **cyclosporine, **dafopriston, *diltiazem, **erythromycin, **fluconazole, **gemfibrozil,**itraconazol, **ketoconazole, **nefazodone, **niacin, **quinupristin, **verapamil} ↑ risk of myopathy or rhabdomyolysis]; *carbamazepine (↓ efficacy); *cholestyramine (↓ efficacy); *colestipol (↓ efficacy); *digoxin (↑ risk digoxin toxicity); *fosphenytoin (↓ efficacy); *phenytoin (↓ efficacy); **protease inhibitors [{amprenavir, atazanavir, indinavir, lopinavir-ritonavir, nelfinavir, ritonavir, saquinavir} (↑ efficacy and risk of myopathy or rhabdomyolysis]; *rifampin (↓ efficacy); *troglitazone (↓ efficacy); *warfarin (↑ risk of bleeding and ↑ risk of rhabdomyolysis).

Food/beverages
*Oat bran (↓ efficacy); *pectin (↓ efficacy); **grapefruit juice (↑ bioavailability (efficacy) and ↑ risk myopathy or rhabdomyolysis.

Incompatible herbs/interaction effect
*St. John's wort (↓ efficacy).

Clinical management
PO; client teaching to report muscle pain, weakness, tenderness, fever, or malaise to healthcare provider immediately. May be taken with food. Do not take with grapefruit juice.

* Severity of reaction indicated by: * moderate, ** severe

spironolactone

Aldactone, Novospiroton

Classification: Selective aldosterone blocker
Therapeutic use: Diuretic, potassium sparing

Incompatible drugs/interaction effect

Aspirin (↓ efficacy); ACE inhibitors [{**benazepril, **captopril, **enalapril, **fosino-pril, **lisinopril, **monopril, **moexpril, **perindopril, **quinapril, **ramipril, **trandolapril} ↑ serum potassium]; angiotensin II receptor antagonists [{**candesartan, **eprosartan, **irbesartan, **losartan, **olmesartan, **telmisartan, **valsartan} ↑ risk of hyperkalemia}]; cyclosporine (↑ hyperkalemia); *digoxin (may ↓ positive inotropic effect, may ↑ serum digoxin level); folic acid (↓ efficacy); lithium (↑ serum lithium levels and risk of toxicity); NSAIDs (↓ diuretic effectiveness, hyperkalemia, ↑ nephrotoxicity); potassium preparations [{potassium acetate, potassium bicarbonate, potassium chloride, potassium citrate, potassium gluconate, potassium iodine, potassium phosphate} risk of severe hyperkalemia], warfarin (↓ anticoagulant efficacy).

Food/beverages

Food increases absorption (↑ efficacy).

Incompatible herbs/interaction effect

Ma huang (↓ hypotensive effect of potassium sparing diuretics); natural licorice (↑ mineralocorticoid activity); yohimbine (↓ diuretic effectiveness).

Lab test interactions

May cause falsely elevated digoxin level. May increase plasma cortisol levels by Mattingly Fluorometric method.

Clinical management

May be taken with or without food. Monitor serum potassium, BUN, and creatinine regularly; provide clients a list of foods high in potassium and stress moderation; advise client to report the following symptoms: immediately irregular heart rate, palpitations, ↓ heart rate, muscle weakness, parenthesias, nausea, and vomiting. Teach client to avoid high-potassium foods: bananas, citrus juices, broccoli, beans, potatoes, spinach, and salt substitutes. With digoxin monitor level (therapeutic range 0.8–2.0 nanograms/mL).

* Severity of reaction indicated by: * moderate, ** severe

vancomycin

Lyphocin, Vancocin, Vancoled

Classification: Miscellaneous

Therapeutic uses: antibiotic, anti-infective

Incompatible drugs/interaction effect

Aspirin, aminoglycosides, cyclosporine, cisplatin, loop diuretics (↑ ototoxic and nephrotoxic effects), metformin (↑ meformin plasma levels); nondepolarizing neuromuscular blocking agents [{atacurium, pancuronium, vecuronium}↑ neuro-muscular blockade]; warfarin (↑ risk of bleeding); ↑ histamine flush when used with general anesthetics in children, vancomycin compatibility with beta-lactam antibiotics is concentration dependent.

Incompatible herbs/interaction effect

↑ CNS depression with kava, valerian, skullcap, chamomile, or hops.

Y-site incompatibility

Albumin, amphotericin B, aztreonam, cefepime, cefotaxime, cefotetan, cefoxitin, ceftazidime, ceftriaxone, cefuroxime, foscarnet, gatifloxacin, heparin, idarubicin, nafcillin, piperacillin/tazobactam, ticarcillin, ticarcillin/clavulanate.

Syringe incompatibility

Heparin.

Lab test interactions

May cause increased BUN levels.

Clinical management

PO; may be taken with food. Dilute with preservative free normal saline. IV administration over at least 60 minutes, rapid infusion precipitates *"red mans syndrome."* Monitor for signs of hearing loss (otoxicity) or decreased urine out-put (neprhotoxicity).

* Severity of reaction indicated by: * moderate, ** severe

Glossary

Absorption – The movement of a drug into the bloodstream.

Additive – A substance that is added to a drug or solution for a combined effect.

Adverse drug reaction (ADR) – Unwanted consequences associated with the use of different drugs.

Agonist – A drug that causes an effect.

Antagonist – A drug that blocks an effect.

Anaphylactic – A severe response to an allergen which can be a drug or other substance.

Antidote – A drug or substance that blocks the action of another drug.

Cross tolerance – When another drug of a similar classification is taken and larger doses are needed to produce the intended effect.

Distribution – Movement of drug molecules within the bloodstream and body tissues where pharmacologic action occurs.

Drug interaction – A reaction that occurs between a drug or other substance that increases or decreases the effect of the other drug.

Drug therapy – The science of using drugs to treat illness, cure disease, and manage an array of symptoms from a multitude of conditions.

Efficacy – A drug's effectiveness in producing therapeutic effects.

Elimination – Elimination of the drug by the body through the kidneys, bowel, lungs, or skin.

Evidence-based – The application of interventions and practice based on research.

Glomerular Filtration Rate (GFR) – Used to determine renal function and is the volume of fluid that is filtered from renal glomerular capillaries into the Bowman's capsule.

Hepatic First Pass – Drugs that are extensively metabolized in the liver where only part of the drug reaches the systemic circulation for distribution to the site of action the first time through.

Hypersensitivity reaction – Occurs when an individual has been previously exposed to a drug or substance and develops antibodies. Additional exposures to the drug or substance may cause signs and symptoms that increase in severity.

Idiosyncratic effect – An unexpected reaction that occurs when a drug is administered the first time.

Metabolism – Process whereby drugs are biotransformed or inactivated within the body.

Pharmacokinetic – The study of the processes where drugs reach their sites of action by absorption, distribution, metabolism, and elimination.

Pharmacodynamic – The drug's action or effects on cells and tissues within the body.

Polypharmacy – Taking a combination of many medications for various ailments in the guise of being helpful. This can sometimes produce detrimental results in a client.

Potency – A drug's strength in producing an effect.

Receptor – The site where drugs interact to produce pharmacological effects.

Therapeutic window/index – The concentration above which the drug is toxic and below which the drug is ineffective.

Tolerance – When the body requires larger doses to produce the same effects.

Toxicity – Occurs when either too much drug is administered or the effects of the drug are increased by another drug or substance to cause adverse effects within the body.

References

Abrams, A.C. (2003) *Clinical Drug Therapy: Rationales for Nursing Practice* (7th edition). Philadelphia: Lippincott Williams & Wilkins.

Abrams, A. C., Pennington, S.S. and Lammon, C. B. (2006) *The Clinical Drug Therapy: Rationales for Nursing Practice* (8th edition). Philadelphia: Lippincott Williams & Wilkins.

"Center for Food-Drug Interaction Research and Education." University of Florida. Available at *www.druginteractioncenter.org*. Accessed November 14, 2006.

Deglin, J. H. and Vallerand, A. H. (2006) *Davis's Drug Guide for Nurses* (10th edition). Philadelphia: F.A. Davis Company.

"Drug Digest." Available at *www.drugdigest.org*. Accessed January 4, 2007.

"Facts about the 2007 National Patient Safety Goals" The Joint Commission. Available at: *www.jointcommission.org/PatientSafety/NationalPatientSafetyGoals/07_npsg_facts.htm*. Accessed January 4, 2007.

"FDA Announces New Prescription Drug Information Format to Improve Patient Safety." United States Food and Drug Administration. Available at: *www.fda.gov/bbs/topics/news/2005/NEW01272.html*. Accessed January 18, 2007.

"FDA Issues Bar Code Regulation." United States Food and Drug Administration. Available at: *www.fda.gov/oc/initiatives/barcode-sadr/fs-barcode.html*. Accessed December 28, 2006.

Guyatt, Gordon and Drummond, Rennie. (2002) *Users' Guides to the Medical Literature: A Manual for Evidence-Based Clinical Practice*. Chicago: AMA Press 706. Kee, J. L. (2004) *Clinical Calculations with Applications to General and Specialty Areas* (5th edition). St Louis, Saunders.

Ostenberg, L. and Blaschke, T. "Medication compliance and avoiding adverse drug reactions." Medscape Today from WebMd. Available at *www.medscape.com/viewarticle/543502*. Accessed November 26, 2006.

"Preventable Adverse Drug Reactions: A Focus on Drug Interactions." Center for Drug Evaluation and Research. Available at *www.fda.gov/cder/drug/drugReactions/default.htm*. Accessed December 27, 2006.

Riedl, M. A. and Casillas, A. M. "Adverse Drug Reactions: Types and Treatment Options." American Family Physician. Available at *www.aafp.org/afp/20031101/1781.html*. Accessed November 30, 2006.

Sackett, D., Rosenberg, W., Gray, J., Haynes, R., and Richardson, W. "Evidence based medicine: what it is and what it isn't." BMJ. Available at *www.bmj.com/cgi/content/full/312/7023/71*. Accessed January 15, 2007.

"Sigma Theta Tau International's Position Statement on Evidence-Based Nursing." Sigma Theta Tau International: Honor Society of Nursing. Available at *www.nursingsociety.org/research/main.html#ebp*. Accessed January 15, 2007.

Springhouse. (2006) *Nursing 2007 Dangerous Drug Interactions*. Philadelphia: Lippincott Williams & Wilkins.

"Strategies to reduce medication errors." United States Food and Drug Administration. Available at *www.fda.gov/fdac/features/2003/303_meds.html*. Accessed December 18, 2006.

"The Merck Manuals." Available at *www.merck.com/mmpe/index.html*. Accessed January 10, 2007.

"Thomson Micromedex." Available at *www.micromedex.com*. Accessed January 4, 2007.

"Top Ten Dangerous Drug Interactions in Long-Term Care." The Multidisciplinary Medication Management Project. Available at *www.scoup.net/M3Project/topten/*. Accessed February 15, 2007.

Trissel, L. A. (2005) *Handbook of Injectable Drugs* (13th edition). Bethesda, MD: Society of Health-System Pharmacists.

Vestal, Christine. "Baby boomers augur old age, new needs." Stateline.org. Available at: *www.stateline.org/live/ViewPage.action?siteNodeId=136&languageId=1&contentId=58924*. Accessed January 4, 2007.

Wilson, B., Shannon, M. T., Shields, K.M., and Stang, C. L. (2007) *Nurse's Drug Guide 2007*. Upper Saddle River, NJ: Prentice-Hall.

Who said nursing can't be fun?

We're the leading "dot calm" resource
when you're feeling stressed.

Check us out 24/7 at
www.stressedoutnurses.com

What will you find there? Along with this
colorful character, you'll see:

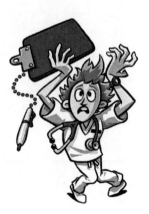

- ✓ **Contests**
- ✓ **Fun, witty articles that will help
relieve your stress**
- ✓ **Resources to help you on your
journey as a nurse**
- ✓ **Much, much more**

So, what are you waiting for?

Get clicking and kiss your stress goodbye!